BEYOND JOGGING . . .
Mike Spino's Fabulous Four-Day Runner's Workshop

Mike Spino is the director of the well-known Esalen Sports Center in California. He is also the creator of unique weekend workshops all around the country that teach runners how to integrate the physical and mental aspects of their sport.

Mike Spino is an expert on the mechanics of running—what breathing and stretching exercises help the most; how to vary your pace; the advantages of different gaits, including the shuffle, the fresh swing and the sprint. But he doesn't stop there. Drawing from the methods of some of the foremost track coaches of the last fifty years, he has designed "innerspace" techniques specifically to help runners discover mind/body running. Based on meditation and mental visualization, these exercises deepen the runner's self-awareness, develop his powers of concentration, increase his relaxation and enjoyment while he runs, and lead him to that ultimate jogging experience—*Runner's High.*

MIKE SPINO'S MIND/BODY RUNNING

Essentia  nce

MIKE SPINO'S MIND/BODY RUNNING PROGRAM

Mike Spino
and
Jeffrey Earl Warren

BANTAM BOOKS
TORONTO · NEW YORK · LONDON

MIKE SPINO'S MIND/BODY RUNNING PROGRAM
A Bantam Book / June 1979

ISBN 0-553-13046-3

Published simultaneously in the United States and Canada

Bantam Books are published by Bantam Books, Inc. Its trade-mark, consisting of the words "Bantam Books" and the por-trayal of a bantam, is Registered in U.S. Patent and Trademark Office and in other countries. Marca Registrada. Bantam Books, Inc., 666 Fifth Avenue, New York, New York 10019.

PRINTED IN THE UNITED STATES OF AMERICA

DESIGNED BY MIERRE

To my mother

M.S.

To Jim McMullen and Janee,
without whom,
New York would never have been possible

J.W.

Contents

I	The Way of the Runner	1
II	The Inner Spaces of Running	13
III	The Zen of Running	25
IV	Visualization Exercises: A Closer Look	42
V	Breathing and Stretching	60
VI	The Physiology of Running Right	93
VII	Variety	114
VIII	Setting Up Your Own Six-Week Program	145
	Appendix	181
	Glossary	196
	Index	207

MIKE SPINO'S MIND/BODY RUNNING PROGRAM

I

The Way of the Runner

We shall not cease from exploration
And the end of all of our exploring
Shall be to arrive again at the beginning
And know the place for the first time.

—T. S. ELIOT

On the face of it, running would seem to be one of the least technical and least mental of all athletic activities. What could be simpler, after all, than going out to a track, a field, or a road and doing what you've been doing naturally ever since you were a child? What physical activity requires less in the way of concentration and mental effort?

Indeed, isn't the naturalness and the simplicity of it the main reason running has become a part of so many millions of Americans' lives over the past several years?

To be sure, its "simplicity" is one of the aspects of running that has made it an important part of my life for so long. However, it's important, I think, that we clarify—and qualify—exactly what we mean by "simplicity." Even more important is getting to the root of what we mean when we use the term "mental" in running.

I realize that most runners don't really give much thought to the mental side of running. Nor do most runners give much thought to the *nature* of their running sessions. Most runners simply *run*. And understandably. If you're like most runners, you run for some very basic reasons. You like the idea of being fit. You enjoy the feeling of well-being that stays with you for hours after a good run. You take pleasure in the feeling of accomplishment that comes from increasing your distances or bettering your times.

I would be the last person in the world to downplay the importance of these motives. Running does keep you fit. It does instill in you a feeling of well-being.

But when I talk about the intellectual dimension of running I'm talking about a dimension that can make the difference between running as something you simply do and enjoy, and running as an experience that can have a profound and beneficial impact on your entire life.

Most runners are unaware of this dimension. Ninety percent of the recreational runners today plod along specific trails or oval tracks, covering their chosen distance at a steady, unvarying pace. On some days they enjoy themselves while running. Often, the workout is pure agony. Peak experiences are few and far between.

I, myself, spent many years as a runner with little awareness of the full dimension of the running experience. Not that I wasn't dedicated to running, and not that I wasn't disciplined. Throughout my teens, I was both. But it wasn't until I came into contact with a number of coaches with imaginative running philosophies, and, later, when I got involved with the Esalen Sports Center in California, that I began to realize that I had much more control than I thought I had over the quality of my running experience. Like you, perhaps, I was one of those runners whose workouts never varied, who would sometimes find a workout pure joy and sometimes find a workout pure agony—one of those runners whose "bad" days outnumbered "good" days but who hung in there because the good days were so very good.

Many recreational runners are skeptical about the importance the mind plays in running. But all great runners know that *running is done with the head, not the legs.* That is why the keystone of my program is based on training the mind to work in positive conjunction with the body. As early as 1961, Dr. J. Kenneth Doherty, the visionary coach at the University of Pennsylvania for many decades, said, "Any sound approach to training for competitive running must plan as deliberately and specifically for the mental aspects of development which precedes or is on an equal basis with the physical aspects of development."

What I learned from my coaches was that it wasn't so much the amount of time and effort you devoted to your running training that counted, it was the specific nature of the training routine. And what I've learned from Esalen, in short, is that the mind is the force that most determines the nature of the running experience. To take training for granted is to waste energy and effort. And to ignore the mind when you run is to not only deprive yourself of much of what running has to offer, it is to limit your capabilities as a runner.

But what exactly am I talking about when I talk about "training" and what do I mean when I talk about using the "mind" in running? These questions aren't simple to answer, but I'd like to try, anyway. First, we'll look at how the way you train (apart from the time and effort you put in) can make a huge difference in your running performance. And then we'll take a look at where the mind fits in.

Training and the Four-Minute Barrier

Everybody knows that it was the Englishman Roger Bannister who first broke the so-called four-minute barrier in the mile run. But few people realize that if it weren't for the development of advanced training techniques, it's likely that the four-minute barrier would still exist today. Even though the average recreational runner is not concerned with improving his time for the mile run, the mile serves as a convenient illustration of how varying techniques have helped runners improve throughout the last half century.

Let's go back to 1913 and to the first great miler of the century, the American John Paul Jones. Jones set the world record that year—4:14.6—but he had little concept of training. He simply ran in a lot of races. The meet was his training ground.

Jones's record was broken in the 1920s by the famous Finn Paulo Nurmi, who in some respects was the first long-distance runner to develop a systematic training routine. Nurmi "trained" by running in the woods, and by working out at different long distances. His method was the forerunner of the training technique known as *fartlek* (the Swedish word for "speed play") that was introduced in the 1940s by the noted Swedish running coach Gosta Holmer.

Holmer developed the concept of fartlek by studying the training methods of the great German 880-yard runner Rudolf Harbig. Harbig was the first man to concentrate on "interval training." He would run short intervals, like 220 yards, as fast as he could. Then he would rest for a period. Run again. Rest. He would then run again until he was exhausted.

What Harbig was doing proved that a runner could get a better "carry," that is maintain a faster speed over a specific distance, by training in this fashion. This method enabled him to set an 880-yard world record—1:46.6—in 1939. He was killed in the war a few years later.

In developing fartlek, Gosta Holmer simply expanded on the concept of interval training. He would map out a 2½-mile course through the woods and have his runners complete the circuit in pairs, running at different gaits and tempos. Instead of running a specific, predetermined distance, like 220 yards, his runners would spontaneously call out a distance (say from here to that tree 40 yards up the trail), and they would cover that distance at a different speed.

Holmer's two most famous protégés, Arne Andersson and Gunder Haegg, used to run this circuit together, calling out different distances. If sprinting is considered as running at 100 percent effort, they might start out at 20 percent effort, but at some point, Arne might say, "Let's run to that rock at 40 percent effort." Once there, they might drop back down to 20 percent. Then Gunder might say, "Let's run 70 percent effort until we reach that fallen log," and Arne might counter by suggesting that they run only 10 percent effort until they reached another arbitrary point.

If this strikes you as a curious way to train, consider the results. In 1944 Andersson ran the mile in 4:01.6 A year later Haegg broke Andersson's record with a 4:01.4.

The question, though, is why? Why were Andersson and Haegg, using a system not much different from the system used by German long-distance runners, able to achieve better times? The answer, I think, lies in the nature of fartlek training as opposed to the much stricter German interval training. The simple fact of calling out distances added a dimension to fartlek training that was missing in the German style of interval training. It added the element of play.

Advancing the Intervals

The 1950s saw the emergence of yet another visionary track coach—the Hungarian Mihaly Igloi. While serving in the Hungarian army, Igloi took three soldiers, Sandor Iharos, Laszlo Tabori, and Istvan Roszavolgy, and working with them, perfected what is considered today the ultimate interval system.

Igloi was very scientific and had little use for spontaneous, playful techniques that Andersson and Haegg had used in the 1940s.

Running, in Igloi's view, was like playing a composition on the violin. If you could master all the different sections of a composition then, in Igloi's judgment, you could put the pieces together, and when the moment of truth arrived, play a perfect concerto.

So Igloi concentrated on putting his runners through long series of short intervals—150 yards, 80 yards, 220 yards—rarely anything over 440 yards. He kept the clock himself and never told the runners what their times were.

Igloi also focused on gaits and efforts. He even gave names to them. He called running at 15 to 50 percent efficiency, for example, a "fresh swing" tempo. "Good swing" was 50 to 80 percent effort, and "hard swing" was 80 to 100 percent effort. "Hard speed" was sprinting. He even had a tempo called "good speed" which was running at good swing tempo but with a different, so-called unnatural motion. At "good speed," Igloi's runners would swing both arms from side to side and let the feet kick out at a 30° angle, imitating the style of a ten-year-old running on a playground. This variation gave weary arm and leg muscles a much needed rest.

In 1955 Igloi's trio broke every major record from 1000 meters to 10,000 meters. In 1956, when the Hungarian revolution broke up this incredible running team, Igloi came to America. Igloi left the U.S. in 1968 and since has coached in Greece. No other coach has produced as many sub-four-minute milers. Probably the most amazing facet of Igloi's career has been his ability to take relatively unknown milers, work with them for a year, and then have these runners, in their first major meet, turn in a sub-four-minute mile. This is precisely what Igloi did with Jim Garrison, who was running a 4:10 mile when he started working with Igloi at the Los Angeles Track Club and ran a sub-four-minute mile a year later.

If you were one of his runners in a training session in which the object was to run four sub-60-second 440s, and if after the third sub-60 440 you felt too exhausted to go on, Igloi wouldn't just order you to "gut it out." Instead, he would have you run a couple of 100s and 150s at fresh swing or good swing tempos.

And when he sensed that your fatigue had passed (and how he could sense this is anybody's guess), he would order a 440 hard swing. Invariably, the altered tempos and intervals would provide you with the rest you needed to run that final sub-60-second 440. "When the body says yes," Igloi would say over and over, "the mind obeys."

Percy Cerutty

While Mihaly Igloi was turning out sub-four-minute milers in California, another coach on the other side of the planet was doing the same thing, but with a much different system. The coach was the Australian Percy Cerutty, whose training method was as far removed from classical interval training as Australia is from Sunset Boulevard.

Unlike Igloi, Cerutty was not particularly scientific. He was a philosopher—a naturalist and an acute observer of nature. If Igloi viewed running as a precise concertolike experience, Cerutty viewed running as an almost cosmic interchange between the runner and his universe. There were no oval cinder tracks in Cerutty's training camps. His runners ran through the woods or on the beaches. They ran barefoot.

Cerutty's first protégé was Roger Bannister's antagonist John Landy. His most famous pupil was Herb Elliott, the most dominating figure in the history of running. Elliott not only lowered the mile record in 1958 from 3:57.2 to 3:54.5, he never lost a mile or a 1500-meter race. And in the 1960 Olympics he won the 1500 meters by the most decisive margin of any race ever run in the Olympics. He retired at 21. There were no more Troys for him to conquer.

What Cerutty did for Elliott was to take him off the hard surfaces and have him run the paths in the forest. For the most part, there were no clockings. The point of training was to enhance Elliott's balance and grace. And Cerutty believed that the best way to develop grace and balance was to run on the uneven terrain of a natural forest.

Cerutty also introduced the concept of "resistance running." He would take Elliott to the beach and have him charge up and down a sand dune. Cerutty also introduced weight lifting as a training technique for long-distance runners.

Probably the most unusual aspect of Cerutty's training philosophy was his psychological approach. Before Elliott would attack a sand dune, for instance, Cerutty would talk to him about St. Francis of Assisi. He would talk about the road to sainthood. About suffering. About surrender. About pain. He'd talk of suffering as the way to inner self-knowledge. Cerutty taught Elliott to be self-reliant, to go to the sand dune on his own and learn to cope with the universe without dependence upon a coach or anyone else. He taught Elliott that pain is not arbitrary, that it can be applied toward a greater sense of accomplishment, that suffering is a part of living, that once it is accepted and not feared, it can be used to help achieve one's destiny.

A student of naturalistic motion, Cerutty wanted his runners to learn from the animals. "Run as the cheetah runs," he used to say. "Stretch as the lion stretches before charging after its prey." The breathing techniques Cerutty developed emulated the movement of wild animals. Even the different running styles he developed— the trot, the amble, the canter, and the gallop—were based on the running motions of animals. Cerutty wanted a runner, literally, to canter, leading with his left forearm, following with the right leg, as though he were a lion romping across the plain.

Cerutty was also keenly aware of the mental strain inherent in running. That's why he insisted on natural settings for his runners. He felt that flowers and animals were important for their distracting effect. They took the mind off pain and fatigue.

So while coaches halfway around the world were clocking their runners in track stadiums, cajoling them to run specific distances in prescribed times, Cerutty was teaching his runners self-reliance, and encouraging them to think about issues of far greater importance than time and distance.

Cerutty did have one famous course which he timed. It was called the Hall Circuit and it was a run through bramble bushes. Like mystics on hot coals, Cerutty's men would charge through that thorny circuit, oblivious to earthly pain. No one has ever approached Elliott's time through the brambles.

Totally dedicated to his students, Cerutty had his own way to get his runners up for a race. When he was coaching Elliott, for example, the two would arrive in town the night before the next evening's race. They'd go to an isolated motel; no fans or reporters were allowed to visit Elliott, for fear they would upset his concentration. Cerutty and Elliott would spend the evening talking not about the next day's race, but about the origin of the universe. Or they might spend hours just sitting in the room together and letting "whatever happens" happen. Cerutty, of course, was oblivious to the concepts of "meditation" or "energy transfer," yet he was a master of these disciplines long before they became fashionable in Western thought.

On the morning of the race Cerutty would take Elliott to a track, where Cerutty would proceed to run himself to total exhaustion. "I am dedicating this run of exhaustion to you," he would tell Elliott. And when he finally regained his breath, he'd turn to Elliott and say, "You may run a faster time tonight than I did, but you will never run harder than I have." Elliott would then proceed to put on one of his patented classical performances.

Arthur Lydiard and Marathon Training

Still another training concept that has become important is the idea known as long continuous distance running, which was developed by Arthur Lydiard, coach of the indomitable Peter Snell. Lydiard believed that if you wanted to run a four-minute mile, you had to prepare yourself by doing 100 miles of long continuous running each week. Lydiard called it marathon training. It is probably the finest way to build up a runner's maximum oxygen intake. Though Long Continuous Distance is perhaps the most popular form of training today, there is much debate as to whether it is the most effective way to train. As you will soon discover, my program places less emphasis on LCD and more emphasis on interval and fartlek training.

The Bill Emmerton Shuffle

One last training concept deserves brief mention. It's known as the shuffle and it was developed by Bill Emmerton, the stunt runner who is forever taking "short" jaunts like, say, from Houston to Cape Kennedy, and doing it in record time. Emmerton is able to run 50 miles a day for 20 days at a time, and the reason he can do it is that he spends much of the time using a shuffling step, a technique I'll explain in detail later.

The Way of the Lung-Goms

The evolution of training techniques over the past 50 years shows pretty clearly, I think, that the nature of a training workout is one of the crucial factors in a runner's performance. True, except for Cerutty's preworkout talks with Elliott, these techniques are not "mental" in the strict sense of the term, but if you want proof of just how *much* a factor the mind can be in running, consider the legendary lung-gom runners of Tibet. This incredible sect of high priests was better known in the 19th century than now, but as recently as the 1930s there were reports of some of them being able to run 600 miles without stopping. Even more remarkably, lung-goms were able to accomplish this mind-staggering feat with *no* prior long-distance training.

How did they do it? Not by jogging around a track, not by running through the picturesque Tibetan mountains, not by charging up sand dunes, and not by running through brambles. They did it by preparing themselves for five years with intensive meditation, coupled with special breathing and stretching exercises. The lung-gom runners, reportedly, would meditate inside wooden barrels. Their powers of concentration were supposedly so strong that they would achieve out-of-body experiences of such intensity that you could hear loud bangs from within the barrel when they "returned" to earth.

The few Westerners who ever witnessed the lung-goms as they ran report that these runners looked as if they were running in a trance and that some of them were actually capable of sleeping while they ran. He does not speak, or look from side to side, but keeps his eyes fixed on a distant object. Apparently, he reaches a point where he does not feel the weight of his own body, and goes on thus for hours without pain or fatigue. It's likely that the physical capabilities of these runners have been somewhat exaggerated, but even if the reports of the distances they were able to cover are only half true, they still stand as powerful testimony to the role that the mind can play in running.

A Program for You

I hope I haven't scared you away with some of these accounts of training systems. You don't have to worry: I'm not going to present you with a program that will force you to meditate in a barrel, charge up sand dunes, and run through brambles. But the training program that you will be introduced to later in this book is based in large part on the concepts that underlie these various techniques.

Basically what I've tried to do is take elements from each of these regimes and develop a series of programs which can benefit you whether you are a recreational or a professional runner.

All of this may sound very complicated, but it's not. For what I've also tried to do is to make the training regimens easy to follow. The whole point of these programs is to make training more enjoyable, less boring, and more productive. If you follow this program you can expect to enjoy yourself more, to have more "peak" experiences when you run. And you can expect to experience less pain, fatigue, and discomfort. Your running distances and your times will improve, but more importantly, the running experience will become more personal, more meaningful, and more enjoyable.

One final word. I recognize how personal running is. No two runners are exactly alike, and not every training regimen is best for every temperament. I doubt, for instance, if the Oxford-bred Bannister, a stickler for neat, orderly schedules, would have broken the four-minute barrier if Cerutty had been his coach, and it's reasonable to assume that Herb Elliott wouldn't have become the runner he became if he had trained under Igloi.

The point is that the ultimate judge of which elements of the training program work best for you is you yourself. I urge you, though, to give yourself a chance with as many as you can. Experiment. Don't prejudge. Give yourself a chance to let running do for you what it is doing for those fortunate runners (and I consider myself one of them) who have found in running an activity that gives added texture, excitement, and meaning to life.

II

The Inner Spaces of Running

In this chapter we're going to look inside ourselves to explore the "inner consciousness" sensations that I consider the true essence of the running experience.

I'm aware that we're heading into some controversial territory. For one thing, the inner experiences of running—the changes in consciousness that take place when you run—are not universal, like the physical changes. Everybody who runs knows what it's like to be fatigued, sore, winded, and stiff; but not everybody who runs experiences a real change in his conscious perception of the outside world or of himself. Many runners, in fact, insist that changes in consciousness are not part of the running experience at all, and that the runners who say they experience a "high" from running imagine a sensation that has no scientific basis. But "runner's high" has been measured and recorded. Researchers, for example, wired Ron Dawes and found that he registered extensive periods of Alpha while running in a marathon. Alpha is a brain wave pattern which indicates an altered state of consciousness, and carries with it measurable physiological changes.

This is another reason why I am not one of the

Doubting Thomases. And scientific evidence aside, I am happy (and grateful) to say that I am not such a runner. Running has provided me with some of the most intense and memorable inner experiences I have ever known—experiences unlike any others I've ever had, experiences so unique they don't lend themselves to conventional description.

But I have not had these experiences because I am special or because I was born with a particular set of genes that makes me more receptive to them. I have had these experiences because my mind is open to them and because I have taken steps in my life to cultivate them. What's more, the kind of experiences I'm talking about are available to anybody—anybody, that is, who is open to them and who is willing to use his or her mind in a way I think the mind should be used for running.

But as biased as I am on this subject, I can understand why some runners deny running's potential to change levels of consciousness. The biggest complaint I hear from beginning runners and from ex-runners isn't about the pain of running but rather the boredom and the monotony of it. And the complaint is understandable. Running can be boring and it can be monotonous.

But it doesn't have to be. Running becomes boring when you run out of habit and duty, and not out of joy. Running becomes boring when your only concern is for the physical aspects: your heart rate, your running times, your injuries. Running becomes boring when you deny yourself access to the total running experience—when you ignore the spiritual aspects of running.

To experience the full dimension of the running experience you have to be open to it. In this chapter, I hope I can make you more open by pointing out some aspects of running and the mind that you may not be aware of.

Running and Meditation

If we are going to talk about altered states of consciousness and running, we have to first talk about—and understand—the phenomenon of meditation. Meditation, as you probably know, is a mental process whose general purpose is to put the mind in a state of calm—a state that would exist all the time were it not for the constant pressures of everyday life and the pressures of our ego-dominated personalities. Not an escape from what we normally think of as reality, meditation is best thought of as a cleansing process that helps you experience life as it actually is, and not as you've been conditioned to see it.

Historically, meditation has never had much impact in the U.S. We are a pragmatic, hard-nosed people. Our characteristic way of achieving inner calm is through external means—material possessions, alcohol, drugs.

In recent years, however, this orientation has begun to change. Popular interest began in 1960, when a mystic from India, the Maharishi Mahesh Yogi, born Mahesh Prasad Varma a.k.a. Maharishi, set up the International Meditation Society in London. That year the Maharishi and his disciples began spreading the word about a technique of meditation known as transcendental meditation, or TM.

The Maharishi, of course, did not invent meditation. Meditation has been a common practice for centuries upon centuries in Eastern cultures and even had a small following in the West. What he did was to popularize a special technique of meditation—one that produces an altered mind state with much less effort and in far less time than had previously been thought possible. You don't have to meditate in a barrel for days or go off to a religious retreat for months. It is a simple matter of setting aside 20 minutes a day, twice a day, and following a simple set of instructions built around the repetition of a simple sound or Sanskrit word.

TM, as everybody knows, became a big success in the U.S., all the more so when books began to verify the fact that measurable changes in body chemistry do indeed take place during meditation—changes in oxygen consumption, in carbon dioxide elimination, in pulse rate, even in blood pressure level.

In his best-selling book *The Relaxation Response,* the Harvard-trained physician and medical researcher Herbert Benson supplied a wealth of empirical evidence to support the position that meditators do, in fact, undergo significant changes in body chemistry—changes whose sum effect is to make them more relaxed. Benson also showed that meditation brings about a substantial increase in the number of so-called alpha waves registered by EEG equipment. Alpha waves are a reflection of a relaxed, balanced internal environment.

The true significance of Benson's findings lie in the fact that they contradict a historical bias among medical people in the U.S. by showing that certain physiological processes thought to be controllable only through the use of drugs could be controlled through meditation.

Meditation and Running

By now you may be wondering what all this talk about meditation has to do with running. Well, it seems that running, under certain conditions, can be a form of meditation too. Running, that is, can produce internal states similar to the internal states that occur during meditation. It would appear to have something to do with the steady, rhythmic movement. This motion presumably has the same repetitive effect on the runner as the mantra has on the meditator. It serves as the calming mechanism that allows the mind to slow down.

This brings up an interesting question. If running embodies these meditative properties, why doesn't it work for everybody? Why don't the majority of runners experience the calming benefits of running? My suspicion is that most runners do not allow it to happen.

Most runners, in fact, prevent it from happening because of their mental approach to running. To explain what I mean, it's necessary to understand a little of how and why we achieve relative states of calm—and how and why we *don't*.

The Physiological Basis of Relaxation

It is never by accident that we feel either anxious or calm: our body is undergoing a specific kind of chemical activity.

The chemical activity isn't going on for its own sake. What we're feeling is an internal bodily response. When we feel anxious and excited, it is a sign that our body is getting stirred up, preparing itself for action— or what scientists are fond of calling the fight or flight response. What we experience as calm is, generally speaking, the absence of fight or flight responses.

The mechanism now believed to be the most responsible for these bodily responses (and the subsequent sensations) is a section of the brain called the hypothalamus. The hypothalamus has the power to activate a number of organs in the body and therefore can control a wide variety of behaviors, including eating, drinking, and even sex.

How does the hypothalamus exert this control? Here is one of the central questions in psychology, and the answer is still being sought. One thing we know is that there is a logic to the hypothalamus's activities. It issues behavioral instructions on the basis of information it receives from other parts of the brain. Our bodies are endowed with an alarm system. The moment any kind of danger is sensed, the hypothalamus gets the signal and immediately activates the sympathetic nervous system. Up goes blood pressure and heart rate. Up goes metabolism. The body is ready for action.

It's a useful system, except for one thing: the system isn't built for abuse. And in today's stress-filled world, abuse is hard to avoid. Many people today live in what may be described as a constant state of inner agitation, their internal machinery in a constant state of action preparedness. But our society allows almost no outlet for these responses, so they remain bottled up.

Death, divorce, inflation, fear of mugging, bumper-to-bumper traffic—you name it, they all put stress on our bodies. This constant diet of stress is now believed to cause many of our most common ailments today, from ulcers to high blood pressure.

All of which brings us back to meditation. One of the main functions of meditation is to produce a state of mind in which the activity of the sympathetic nervous system is reduced and the entire nervous system is tidier—better balanced. Meditation doesn't change the outside world, mind you. It simply changes the way in which your body is responding. Since much of what we're responding to doesn't present any real and immediate danger to our survival anyway, we're better off. The precise means by which meditation quiets the hypothalamus isn't known, but recent research suggests that the answer lies in the activity of certain chemical substances known as neurotransmitters—chiefly norepinephrine. Meditation appears to cut down on the amount of norepinephrine flowing through the nervous system; thus it slows down sympathetic nervous system activity.

The Role of Mental Attitude in Running

We've been talking more about meditation and relaxation than we have about running. Now it's time to look into the kind of mental approach to running that can allow you to experience the calming effect that some runners enjoy.

Let's look, first of all, at what may be preventing us from experiencing this calming effect. One obvious problem is that the physical demands of running put the body in an active, energized state. Talking about achieving a sense of calm while we run is, in a sense, a contradiction in terms. For this reason, you can't expect a meditationlike reaction to occur when you run if you don't take certain steps to help the reaction along.

This brings up the crucial question: *How should*

you try to manage your mind during a run so that you can achieve inner experiences similar to those you might receive if you were to meditate?

An obvious answer might be to practice a form of transcendental meditation while you run—that is, to chant. But I do not recommend TM as a meditation form for runners while running. The problem with TM is that it tends to put you out of contact with your body, and as we saw in the last chapter, it's important that you recognize what your body is saying throughout a run.

Is there an alternative? I think there is. The alternative is Zen meditation.

Zen Meditation

If you came to one of my workshops, you would soon discover that I spend as much time training your mind as I do your legs.

I try to conduct my workshops loosely along the lines of a Zen center, but this is not to say that my students shave their heads and don white robes. My students come from every stratum of American life—from the unemployed to the overpaid. They bring to my workshops a variety of motivations. About the only thing they have in common is a love of running, and a vague quest for guidance in their search for the inner knowledge and hidden truths running can show them.

My choice of Zen meditation as the form best used when running has not been made arbitrarily. Perhaps you'll appreciate why I made this choice once you understand what Zen is.

Zen is a Japanese word meaning "meditation." It began as *dhyana* in Sanskrit, migrated to China and became *ch'an,* and arrived in Japan as *Zen.*

The chief difference between Zen meditation and other meditative disciplines, such as TM, lies in the mental approach. The essense of TM is concentration on one point—a mantra—and in this way erasing the confusing activities of daily life and allowing a calm, passive attitude to arise.

Zen, on the other hand, is more concerned with what can be called detached awareness. The central concept of Zen is a *focused attention* (as opposed to single-minded concentration) on what Zen masters refer to as the "here and now." Zen is a form of awareness meditation. As Chogyam Trungpa explains in *Meditation in Action* (Berkeley, Calif., 1970):

> In this kind of meditation practice, the concept of *nowness* plays an important part. In fact, it is the essence of meditation. Whatever one does, whatever one tries to practice, is not aimed at achieving a higher state or at following some theory or ideal, but simply without any object or ambition trying to see what is *here and now*. One has to become aware of the present moment through such means as concentrating on the breathing, a practice which has been developed in the Buddhist tradition. This is based on developing the knowledge of nowness, for *each respiration is unique, it is an expression of now*. Each breath is separate from the next and is fully seen and fully felt, not as a visualized form or simply as an aid to concentration, but it should be fully and properly dealt with.

It's reasonable to wonder about the differences in body responses between Zen meditators and yoga meditators (the name used for mantra meditators). And differences there are.

When researchers wired up meditators and compared the yogis to the Zen people, they found that both yogic meditators and those practicing *zazen* ("Zen meditation") tended to have slower heart rates, take fewer breaths, and register a decreased level of oxygen consumption (slowed metabolism). High incidents of alpha activity were apparent in both groups.

But when the experimenters tried to interrupt concentration (alpha states), the yogis registered very few "alpha blocks." So intent on their mantras were the yogis that they didn't notice the outside stimuli foisted upon them by the researchers. To break their concentration, researchers flashed lights, made loud noises, even touched their skin with hot glass tubes, but to no avail. The yogis maintained alpha.

Those practicing zazen, on the other hand, consistently showed alpha blocks, which is to say that as soon as an outside stimulus, like a loud bang, arose, the zazen meditators would register an alpha block for 3 to 5 seconds. This is exactly what happens to ordinary people who try to attain alpha during meditation: alpha blocks appear at the slightest interruption to their concentration. The difference though, is that while ordinary people have difficulty returning to the alpha state, zazen meditators return *immediately*. Their pattern of alpha blocking is proof of their spectacular ability to "be here now."

But Zen is an incredibly involved and complicated discipline. You could spend a lifetime and not understand it fully. A Zen master put it this way, "It is as complex as a bowl of rice, and as simple as the cosmos."

Perhaps this well-known story sums it up: Two students meet on the road. One says, "My master is so magnificent that I can stand on one side of the river, hold up a scroll, and though he stands on the other side of the river, my master writes on my scroll."

The second student says, "My master is so magnificent that he eats when he's hungry and drinks when he's thirsty."

In other words, the second student's master has learned to live absolutely in the present, without concern for the past or future. He is experiencing absolute samadhi.

The Runner as Zen Meditator

"Every once in a while, when I'm running, I feel a sense of tremendous well-being come over me. Everything about me feels in harmony. I feel smooth, and my breathing is so relaxed that I get the feeling I can run forever. I'm not aware of time or space—only a remarkable sense of calm."

This is how one runner I know describes the phenomenon known as "runner's high." Maybe you've had
a variation of the same experience. I know I have. It's
a euphoria unlike anything else you can experience.
Your mind is void of any unpleasant thoughts. Time
seems to slow down, and it's as if your entire body is
enveloped with contentment. You are intensely aware
of yourself, yet you feel unified with everything around
you. You feel lighter than air, and on occasion you feel
as if your mind is out in space somewhere, watching
your body run. And it is during these moments that
you experience what Zen masters call the sense of
samadhi.

To achieve samadhi is the goal of every Zen meditator, and it should be the goal of every runner as
well. Samadhi is the reaching of a transcendent com-
munion with the deepest levels of your inner self.

This is not to say that you can attain absolute samadhi the first time you run. You may never attain it.
But that's not the point of your meditation. You meditate not to reach samadhi, but to approach it. Few
activities in your everyday life will give you even a
hint of samadhi. On the other hand, there may have
been times in your life when you have experienced a
kind of samadhi without being aware (afterward) that
you were in the state.

In absolute samadhi time ceases to exist because
there is no past or future—only present time. In
everyday life, this timelessness is experienced usually
only during moments of great happiness or great crisis.

It happens when you are young and in love, but
have to be in by midnight. You glance at your watch
and see that it is only eight o'clock. You rejoice that
you have four whole hours before you have to leave
each other. Twenty minutes later you check your watch,
and it reads 12:15! It can't be! You haven't been together more than 20 minutes, yet your watch says that
you're already late getting home.

What has happened, of course, is that you and the
person you love were so absorbed in each other, so alert
to every blinking of each other's eyes, that you were

in veritable samadhi—your psychological time was reduced to practically nothing. You were so taken with your young lover that there was no "self" (reflecting) consciousness. Your ego was negated. Your thoughts were negated. You weren't aware of your own actions.

Katsuki Sekida (in *Zen Training, Methods and Philosophy,* p. 121) refers to "psychological time," and how events such as great happiness or catastrophe affect its duration:

> . . . we may deduce that psychological time is created by the frequency of operation of the reflection action of consciousness. In our ordinary life there is an average frequency of this action and we can roughly estimate by long experience that a certain feeling of frequency corresponds to an hour of physical time. However, in extreme circumstances, when the reflecting action of consciousness fails to operate, our estimates fall short and an hour seems like five minutes.
>
> Time completely disappears in absolute samadhi, and so does space. Causation also disappears. There is only a row of events. This state of no time, no space, and no causation is simply realized, without discussion, as an immediate experience in absolute samadhi.

If that last paragraph were paraphrased and included the words "runner's high," wouldn't you think you were reading a first person account in some runner's magazine?

Indeed with a few words changed here and there, the quotation is a fairly adequate description of runner's high. The problem for most runners, though, is that their experience with runner's high is random and erratic. It comes and goes (mostly goes) when least expected, and it seems to visit your psyche so rarely that if you run to experience runner's high, it's hardly worth the effort.

Most runners who experience what they take for runner's high are so delighted by this transcendent experience, they immediately go out and try to recapture it. In doing so, they miss the point entirely, for no two transcendent experiences are the same. You can never recapture what *was* in Zen, and never experience what you set out to experience. You can only experience the moment at hand. To experience this moment in the moment is the "high" you can experience as a runner.

What it comes down to is this. Despite what many runners may tell you, there is a transcendent state that can come from running. We know this not only from the personal accounts of runners who've experienced this state but from the similarity of these accounts with the accounts of transcendent experiences offered by students of Eastern religions. We know this, too, because recent experiments have shown that runners who've been wired up by researchers demonstrate similar physiological adaptations to the adaptations shown by yogis—adaptations that scientists are now willing to acknowledge are commensurate with altered states of consciousness.

Once you acknowledge the possibility of experiencing this high, you enhance the chances of your having the experience. Then it becomes a matter of the quality of the experience. You'll know it when it comes. As Robert Pirsig points out, in *Zen and the Art of Motorcycle Maintenance,* quality may be difficult to define but you know it when you see it or experience it.

III

The Zen of Running

The mind can be trained to do one of two things for you in a run: it can take your attention away from the experience, or it can intensify the attention you give to the run. Here, essentially, is the difference between what might be called the trancendental meditation approach to running and the Zen approach.

It might seem that the yogic approach to meditation would be better suited for running than the Zen approach. After all, aren't pain and boredom the two biggest problems that face most runners? And isn't the purpose of yogic meditation to take you away from these sensations through intense concentration? Isn't it true, too, that the feature of running many people—particularly highly charged executives—like most is its ability to clear the head? "If I have a big problem I'm trying to solve," an executive at one of my workshops once told me, "the best thing I can do for myself is to go out and run. Somehow, during the run I always get a perspective that I didn't have before."

I'm not surprised running induces the kind of mental calm that gives us a fresh, less cluttered perspective on our problems. I do *not*, however, recommend that you consciously mull over your problems as you run. It's simply that, if you have something on your mind, the solution may often pop up spontaneously as you run.

And one of the beauties of Zen (or any other meditation form) is that you don't have to believe in it for it to work. All you have to do is practice the discipline. They say, if you practice meditation long enough, in time, *quantity will become quality*.

Neither am I surprised to hear from runners who know nothing about yogic meditation or Zen (and couldn't care less) but still report a sensation that can legitimately be called runner's high. What happens, I think, is that a person who runs regularly brings about, without trying, a balanced integration of mind and body that is in effect the kind of mental state sought by meditators.

Why, then, do I advocate a Zen approach to running?

The main reason, I suppose, has to do with my attitude toward not only running but life itself. There is something about going out of your way to take your mind off some present experience that strikes me as being a very unnatural way to live. It's a little like a scene in the movie *Getting Straight,* in which Elliott Gould's staying powers are complimented by a woman he's just gone to bed with. "It was nothing," he said. "I just had to replay the entire 1954 World Series to do it."

To take your mind away from the moment at hand when you run seems no different to me from thinking about the 1954 World Series when you're in bed with someone you love. True, it may "improve" your performance. But what are we talking about when we talk about improved performance? Is missing out on the totality of the experience a fair price to pay for improvement? Not in my judgment.

Zen is different. Zen strives to put you *into* the moment—to make you superaware of your every experience—not in relationship to past or future experiences, but as it is happening at this moment . . . now.

Becoming a Zen Runner

Since it takes years of concentrated study to become a Zen master, you have every right to wonder about the practicality of Zen to the average runner. Let me put your mind to rest. You're not going to master Zen by reading this book or by attending a workshop or two. But you can incorporate some of the techniques of Zen into your daily running routine, and moreover, you can start to think of your running more along the lines of a Zenlike experience.

Why? Two reasons. First, adopting a Zenlike approach to running will enable you to discover facets of yourself you didn't know about: it will intensify your sense of self-awareness (not to be confused with self-consciousness). More to the point, a Zenlike approach to running will improve the quality of your running experience. It will give you a runner's high superior in quality to any you may have experienced. It will do this because you will not only experience the psychological and physiological changes that are the inherent features of an altered state of consciousness, but *will directly perceive the experience of the run itself*. You will be aware of your breathing, for example, as an experience. You will be more keenly aware of everything you see when you run—each tree, each slope, each change in the landscape. The sun, the tree, the road, and yes, even the pain in your side—they'll be one and yet all be separate at the same time.

The poet W. B. Yeats asked how could anyone separate the dancer from the dance. He could just as well have been talking about separating the runner from the run. When the run becomes a thing of strength, grace, and synchronized beauty, can you, the runner, be anything less?

I keep thinking about Herb Elliott, who more than any other competitive runner ran as a form of self-expression. When Elliott won the Olympic gold medal by running the 1500 meters in 3:35.6, there was not another runner within 40 yards of him when he crossed the finish line. Elliott didn't need to be pushed in order to run his fastest. He didn't need another runner to egg him on to greatness. He did it by himself, and for himself.

Other runners have recorded faster times than Elliott, but none has approached his depth. Most distance runners today get by on sheer physiological talent and on a mindless, almost fascistic sort of dedication. Theirs is a one-dimensional talent, embodying none of the emotional intensity that Elliott was able to generate.

You have probably encountered many such runners (though on a less grand scale) yourself: wooden runners who experience nothing but a crazed obsession to run faster and longer. Runners whose talk is all of pulse beats, lap times, miles per week. Runners who lack any degree of spiritual wholeness, who run dead, in effect. These are runners who care little about the richness of the running experience, runners who hate running but feel they have to do it.

Be wary of such people. Chances are, they will mock the spiritual aspects of running—and not just of running, but of life in general. They mock because they don't understand what a spiritual experience is, and are afraid of what they don't understand. If you spend too much time with them, you'll start to feel and act the same way. As the sages say, if you walk with a lame man for a year, you will start to limp too.

But what about the pain of running, and the boredom of running? How do you ease their negative impact by intensifying your interaction with them? Do you reduce the pain of a hot pot handle by holding on to it longer?

Not quite. But what you must do first is to accept the reality of pain and boredom as an inherent part of running. Second, don't expect the intense psychic pleasures of running to come daily. I don't care how Zenlike your approach to running is, you are going to experience pain or boredom, and there will be runs where you will experience both.

So don't misunderstand me. I do not glorify the pain and drudgery of running. And I'm not going to convince you that if you don't enjoy the unpleasant aspects of running, you are somehow spiritually deficient. No. Enjoyment of these things is not what we're after, but the acceptance of them—true acceptance of them—as part of the total running and total athletic experience. You'll never eliminate them, but there is much you can do to minimize their negative impact. I'm not talking about gimmicks or wonder cures. I'm talking about mental techniques that can be developed and improved on—techniques that will help you work *with* pain and boredom and hold them in abeyance so that their presence in the running experience is the exception and not the rule.

Basic Zen Breathing

Probably the most basic of all Zen exercises is a simple one that involves nothing more than counting breaths. This exercise is to Zen what chanting the mantra is to TM.

The TMers also work to still the mind. They do it by using a mantra. Zen favors the counting of breaths and the watching of thoughts.

When counting breaths, you start by counting the inhalations and exhalations. Count "One" as you inhale and say "Two" as you exhale. Do this until you reach ten, and then repeat. Say the words to yourself. Try to concentrate on the breaths. See each breath as an individual occurrence. Try to breathe from your diaphragm.

After a few minutes of counting each inhalation and exhalation, try counting your exhalations only. This takes more concentration. Say nothing as you inhale, but count from one to ten as you exhale. If you lose track because your mind wanders, don't fret. Just go back to one and start over again.

Expect your mind to wander at first. And when it does, passively observe those thoughts and return to the counting of the breaths.

This Zen exercise should be practiced twice a day for about 20 minutes. Ideally you should try to meditate immediately before or after a run, but it is important to try to establish a regular meditation practice. The more regularly you meditate, the easier it becomes.

Counting of breaths allows you above all to begin observing your thoughts, watching what actually passes through your mind. Don't worry when your thoughts seem disjointed and sometimes nonsensical. Watch them. Pay attention. Pay closer attention. Try to slow them down. Try to drop one of those thoughts. Yes, *drop* it from your consciousness. If thoughts appear between the counting of breaths, watch them closely. Try to stop one of them. Try to stop a specific thought, like a freeze frame from a motion-picture camera. Zen masters say that if you can stop all thoughts for 7 seconds you will enter satori, one of the steps on the way to samadhi. If you can discipline yourself to stop thoughts for 11 minutes, you will reach samadhi.

How to Use Zen When You Run

One of the best features of Zen is that you don't have to devote your life to it in order to get something out of it. At my workshops, my goal is not to train Zen masters. It's to create an awareness of how a Zenlike approach to running can enrich the experience. So let's look at how Zen can help you deal with the aspects of running that most runners find especially troublesome: pain and boredom.

Pain

It is impossible to talk about running without getting into the subject of pain, but pain is a tricky subject to discuss. Aldous Huxley was fond of quoting a yogi friend who said, "Pain is a matter of opinion."

The ability of yogis to withstand pain is, of course, well known. And if you talk to professional and college football players you can understand how relative pain is. Most professional athletes differentiate between pain and injury. You play with pain. Only if you're injured (read: "near death") do you sit out a game.

Runners often talk in terms of "pain one" and "pain two." Pain one is the minor pain, like the soreness you get in your calf after a fairly long run. Your calf hurts the next day, but you can run on it, working the pain out, without doing further damage. But pain two is severe pain: what you feel when you break something or pull a muscle or a tendon. Try to gut this kind of an injury and run on it, and you're likely to make the injury far more serious.

But how do you differentiate between pain one and pain two? How do you tell the difference between the pain from a serious injury and a pain that is mostly in your head? This is a complicated question, since you can't ignore the psychological component of pain. A toothache, for example, hurts a lot more when you think it means that a wisdom tooth has to come out than when the pain represents the expected aftermath of a treatment you've already received. Most of us can endure severe pain for short periods—as long as we know it's going to end soon. It's the pain whose end we can't predict that gives us the most trouble.

Running with Pain

Here is the situation. You're running along your usual route one morning when you get hit with a sharp pain in the lower part of your leg. What should you do? Stop? Ignore the pain? Run on? Well, let me tell you what I would do. If the pain were of a kind I'd never experienced, I'd play it safe. I'd stop running and take a closer look. I'd flex my leg carefully to see whether the pain intensified. I'd put gradual pressure on it. If the pain eased, I might continue the workout, but I'd keep alert to the pain. I don't want to aggravate an injury, especially an injury I don't understand.

On the other hand, if the pain is a familiar pain—a sign of an old injury, perhaps, or from lactic acid buildup, my approach would be different. I might ease up a little, but I probably wouldn't quit running—as long as the pain didn't become too unbearable.

An experienced runner who knows his or her body

and knows how the body functions during a run is much better off when it comes to pain than an inexperienced runner, or an experienced runner who's never taken the time to look into such matters as lactic acid buildup. (An experienced runner who knows his body knows that the pain being created by a lactic acid build-up will disappear as soon as the lactic acid gets recycled.) When in doubt, however, follow the runners' maxim: "Train, don't strain."

But even experienced runners have trouble differentiating between "real" and "imagined" pain. Let's look into this.

The Mental Side of Pain

Once when he was running in a 10,000-meter race, Michael Murphy, the founder of the Esalen Institute, recalls that he was floating along in a smooth, harmonic fashion when it suddenly occurred to him that he was one of the leaders. This unexpected discovery pleased him and he remembers smiling to himself. But seconds later he was hit with the first major stomach cramp of his running career. He couldn't shake it. He finished the race, but he finished in a great deal of pain.

Michael explained the phenomenon as "devil thought." Just thinking that conscious thought—even though it wasn't a negative thought—was enough to throw his harmonious, totally integrated mind/body system out of whack.

What happened to Murphy that day is not unlike what happens to people in biofeedback sessions when they see the light that informs them they're in alpha. "I've got it," they shout, only to discover that as soon as they make the announcement, the light goes out. "A moment's thought is but passion's passing bell," as John Keats once put it.

You can't separate your mental and emotional state from your physiological state. Granted, what happened to Michael Murphy (a positive thought causing physical discomfort) is something of a rarity. Not so rare is a cramp that arises because of negative inputs into consciousness. Professional tennis players will tell you that a sore arm hurts a lot more when you're losing or worried about losing than when you're on your way to an easy win. I am certain that if you talk to professional runners, you'll find that they suffer the most discomfort on days when they are not in a positive frame of mind.

This is a roundabout way of explaining why it is so useful and important for you, as a runner, to pay close attention to your thoughts as you run. That doesn't mean you control your thoughts, or oversee them like a prison guard with a high-powered rifle. The trick is to keep a Zenlike slight detached awareness going, keeping a watchful mental eye on all thoughts, positive and negative.

Here's an example. You're running along on a normal day with the usual quick succession of thoughts racing through your mind. You have a date with someone you like that evening. The sunset looks nice. You remember a lovely sunset you saw on a trip a few years ago. But the trip brings to mind the fact that you haven't started saving for this year's vacation yet, and what's more, may not be able to save any money.

At this moment you may feel a slight twinge in your side, or maybe your knee. If you're an experienced thought watcher, you'll go back in your mind and figure out which thought may have triggered the pain. And if you are schooled in the art of thought watching, you'll be able to replace that negative thought with a positive thought.

I said "replace" the thought. "Replace" underscores the fact that you can't repress or expunge a negative thought. You can't force yourself *not* to think negative thoughts. (This will only produce a climate conducive to more negative thoughts.) You go with the thought, replacing the negative thought with a positive one, but doing it without force.

The ability to isolate negative thoughts and replace them is not a simple trick, but it's something that people who meditate often find relatively easy. Meditation gives you some degree of mastery over what does and doesn't enter your consciousness.

Even if you can't drop or replace the negative thought, recognizing the source of the negative feedback often has the effect of neutralizing the thought and of driving the pain away.

We're not talking about pain from an actual injury—a sprain or a pull. We're talking about the broad category sometimes referred to as psychosomatic pain. Psychological induction is often the reason that a chronic injury that usually causes mild pain suddenly generates severe pain. I don't want to give the impression that isolating negative thoughts is going to make you oblivious to the pain caused by a sprained ankle or a bad knee. But being able to use your thoughts during a run is an enormously valuable tool in running. One of the keys toward developing this mastery lies in the development of the mental skill of visualization.

Using Visualization

Visualization is a mental technique that isn't really related to Zen but can be used with Zen techniques to cope with some of the difficulties of running. Visualization is nothing more than running with a preplanned picture in your mind. The lung-gom walkers, for example, visualized that they were running to a "distant star." And more and more athletes today, baseball players and tennis players in particular, are using visualization techniques to help them maintain consistent performance under pressure.

I have found visualization enormously effective in overcoming boredom and fatigue and in minimizing pain. I've created a series of visualizations for my workshops that I believe can work for most runners. I'll describe some of them later, but first let me describe one that is very useful in helping you determine whether a pain represents a definite injury or is the result of a negative thought flow.

This visualization works on the premise that if you can distract your mind from pain, the body will find out for itself if the injury is real. Let's assume you have a pain in your upper leg that keeps coming and going, and you can't tell if you've got an injury there or not. Here's what to do.

1. Stand still with your eyes closed.

2. Picture a circle that is blank in the middle but has a thick rim. **O**

3. Fill in the circle with black. **●**

4. Now envision a white circle with a black dot in the middle. **⊙**

Follow these four steps before you start to run again, first with your eyes closed, then with "soft eyes" (your eyes open just wide enough so you can see where you're going).

Now you're ready to run.

If while you are running the thought of the injury comes to mind, use "soft eyes" visualization, picturing first the lined circle, filling the circle with black, and then visualizing the white circle with a dot in the middle. Each time the injury comes back to mind, force it out by visualization. Your goal is to use the visualization to keep the thought of the real or imagined injury from entering your mind. If you can relax while doing this visualization, "imagined" pain will not interfere with your run, but a real pain will persist.

Advanced Zen and Pain

I mention the following Zen technique with a good deal of reservation. The problem is that if you are an inexperienced runner or an inexperienced Zen meditator, you could wind up in a hospital.

This technique of dealing with pain is rooted in the basic Zen notion that if you can stay in the moment, without past, without future, you can live through almost anything, even the worst torture.

There's only one catch. The realization must be authentic—not feigned. You stay in the moment not to beat the pain, but to experience life. That pain at that moment is you. It is your destiny, your unique form of living.

Let's say you're running in a 10-mile race and about three-quarters of the way through you feel yourself becoming nauseated. Soon pain sets in.

If you can surrender (yes, surrender) to the situation, and in surrendering give up the result and long only to fully know the uneasiness of your situation, the run will become spiritual, not painful for you. You may have to close your eyes for an instant (but without falling or losing balance), in order to go "inside" yourself, there to observe your movements, noticing that you are not going *that* fast, getting accustomed to the unfamiliar feeling, making it part of you.

If you stay in this state, the finish line will loom and you will pour into the run, galloping with abandon toward the finish—not despite the pain but *with* the pain, which at this point isn't pain at all but simply you.

A little heavy? Perhaps. Still, the point is that while pain is not fun, it is not to be feared. It can be observed, understood, and ultimately conquered.

Boredom

If it were possible for us to stay in the moment totally, boredom would cease to exist. Not even the most advanced Zen student is capable of living a life entirely free of boredom, so it doesn't make sense to expect as much from the recreational runner.

Boredom is a problem all runners face. Some runners simply handle it better than others, just as some people deal with boredom better in everyday life.

Cicero said, "Never less alone than when wholly alone." With such an attitude he would have made a great marathoner. Unfortunately, most of us are not accustomed to thinking this way. We fear loneliness and avoid solitude. Our culture has not taught us how to cultivate being alone, and we are not trained to deal with it. Our way of dealing with voids is to fill them with outside stimuli. When we clean house, we rarely devote full attention to the work at hand. We put on the radio or the TV. We spend more time reading editorials than we do writing down our own thoughts. Indeed, how many people do you know who have taken the time to have a conversation with themselves?

Our normal pattern is not to pay attention to the activity we are engaged in. A teenager watches "Charlie's Angels" while doing Algebra II homework or a Romeo thinks about the 1954 World Series while making love. Our culture has conditioned us to rely on other people and outside events to provide our entertainment, to provide our thoughts, to provide our feelings. What we lack most in this country is something beyond material needs: psychic self-sufficiency.

Happily the situation appears to be changing, and the popularity of running is a tremendously positive symptom that we may be turning back the tide of psychic dependency. Running is almost entirely an individual activity. I say "almost," because even running is in danger of being swallowed up by our frantic drive to belong. Running clubs are popping up all over, and corporations are beginning to sponsor running teams in the fun runs. In certain communities, some tracks and areas of city parks are more "in" than others. These invidious group encroachments on a purely individualistic activity are just another sign of our unwillingness, or unpreparedness, to be alone.

I don't condemn these trends, but I think there's a danger in them. As I have been saying all along, the ultimate reward of running lies in its spirituality—the opportunity it gives you to know yourself. But you can't realize this benefit unless you experience the solitary aspect of it. Don't brood about the loneliness: rejoice in it. What's wrong with being by yourself? After all, how can you expect others to want to be around you if you don't want to be left alone with yourself for, say, an hour each day? Use your running as an opportunity to get acquainted with yourself. Experiment with your mind and body. Pay attention. Be *in* the moment. Watch how your body reacts under various conditions. Watch what thoughts emerge from your unencumbered mind. Create your own world, as a child, alone in a sandbox, creates an inpenetrable world, free from the tyranny of adults and his peers.

OK, so you dread workouts. Fake it for a while. Yes, fake it. Pretend you like them. Pretend to look forward to them. Pretend to be glad to finally be alone for a while. You will be amazed at what a positive attitude can do to a negative mental state. And running is a curious activity. After a while, quantity becomes quality.

Of course, it's going to take time to change your mental attitude—so do it gradually rather than giving up running because you are bored or because you don't like the solitude of it. And if it's too much for you that you are alone, find a good running mate.

As for the boredom of running itself, the programs presented later in this book are designed in large part to reduce it. The sheer variety of the workouts should go a long way to reduce boredom. Instead of plodding around the same track for the same distance at the same speed, day after day after day, you will be doing something different and fresh every day. New experiences. New challenges.

But different workouts each day and even a running partner will not eliminate boredom entirely. Unfortunately, as I said earlier, few of us are sufficiently adept at being constantly in the Zen sense of the here and now. That's why I advocate a number of mental exercises that you can do while running, while meditating, and during recovery periods after a run. I call them running visualizations.

Running visualizations work best during intervals, or for short burst of times during long runs. They're not difficult to do, but you have to work at them. You have to use your mind.

Forming Mental Pictures

Let's start our look into visualizations by talking about how to form a picture in the mind. Let's suppose you're outside, and you hear a bird chirping. Close your eyes and imagine what the chirping bird looks like. Then open your eyes slightly—just enough so that if you were running you could see where you were going, but not so wide that you lose the mental picture. This is the "soft eyed" technique mentioned earlier. Soft eyes is one of the basic tools in visualization.

One of the most effective boredom-alleviating visualizations is the "big hand." Begin by picturing a large hand coming down from the sky. Then concentrate on the hand. What does it look like? Is it wrinkled? Can you see the veins in the back of the hand? Try to actually feel the top of the hand touching your neck—feel the fingers pressing into the small of your back. With this image firmly planted into your mind, you begin your interval, giving yourself over to the power of the hand, letting the hand, not legs, take you across the field.

Another useful visualization for boredom is the "rope tow." Imagine a harness around your waist with a rope attached from it to a rock or a tree somewhere in the distance. Then as you run, imagine yourself being reeled in, allowing the rope to do all the work.

These are just two of the many visualizations you can do while running. A little imagination and you can create many others that are tailored to your personality. You might prefer to envision yourself as a spinnaker on a sailboat, or a genie riding on a magic carpet. Be inventive; but be thorough. The more detailed your visualization is, the easier your run will be. The reason is that as you concentrate on visualizing, you free your physical body to relax and run in an unencumbered way. Boredom, remember, is an unpleasant experience. Its physical effect is to tense up certain muscle groups, and the tenseness makes the running harder and only increases the feelings of boredom. The circle never ends.

On the other hand, as your mind concentrates on the visualization, it forgets about boredom, allowing muscles to relax. This, in turn, makes the run more effortless, more enjoyable, less boring, . . . get the picture? If you are going to get caught in a cycle, why not make it a pleasurable, positive one?

Moving visualizations are not the only ones useful to the runner. In the next chapter I'll describe a number of important standing visualizations. They deal with energy transfer and the process of recharging yourself through psychic self-regulation, both during a workout and afterward. I will also list four guided fantasies. A guided fantasy is a story line with a universal application. It describes a set of information that will work similarly for many people. The four fantasies have been used hundreds of times in my workshops to break the social ice, open the imagination, and help people become more aware of their physicality. The fantasies work well in the short term, and are especially effective in a long-range meditation program.

In guided fantasy you are lulled into the suggestion of a story line which has gaps. Your responsibility is to fill in the gaps with your imagination, let yourself flow with the fantasy. You may want to read the fantasies on a tape recorder, and play them back to yourself—or have another person read them to you. Using them to supplement your meditations can bring long-lasting rewards.

Relaxation Through Visualization

"I must have faith in my body and allow it to run instinctively without the mind," Herb Elliott writes in *The Golden Mile.* "In races I must let my body go—relax one hundred percent."

We've been talking about controlling the mind. But "control" is a loaded word. As Elliott's comment indicates, the ultimate goal of a runner should be to run instinctively—"without the mind."

If it all seems contradictory to you, don't worry. It *is* contradictory in many respects, and reflects the dilemma faced by all beginning Zen students: the problem of trying not to try. Zen meditation is a mental discipline whose purpose is to free you from your mind—

to remove the judgmental mind from the experience and allow you to make direct connections with the here and now. But the problem with any discipline—mental or not—is that there is always a tendency to force things—to make things happen.

I mention this by way of summarizing what we've gone over up until this point in this chapter. Apart from whatever spiritual rewards a Zen approach to running can bring, it produces a state of body and mind that is central to the success of just about any activity. I'm talking about relaxation. There is no longer any scientific question about the matter. Anxiety and other negative mental states create tension in the body, and tension inhibits performance.

How do you achieve the balance? How do you strive for goals, compete, work to improve yourself, withstand pain and boredom—and do all of these things in a relaxed state of mind?

I don't pretend to hold the answer to this question. There are no *real* answers in Zen, only searches for answers and occasional flashes of enlightenment.

But the balance is there to be achieved and experienced. I know because I've experienced it—not regularly but enough so that each time I run I'm motivated to make the search again.

This is all I can promise you. There is no six-week program to enlightenment, and there is no one right way to self-knowledge. What I've tried to do in the last two chapters is present you with some of the basic principles of Zen and show you how these principles relate specifically to the running experience. Applying these principles to your running may not lead you to enlightenment, but I feel safe in saying that it will give you a new perspective on running, and a new perspective on yourself.

IV

Visualization Exercises:
A Closer Look

Being aware of a concept, and even believing in the concept, is not enough to guarantee that the concept will work for you. If the ideas I've talked about in the last two chapters are going to have impact on your running and your life, you're going to have to work with them, to practice them.

In this chapter I describe a number of mental exercises and mental visualizations designed to help you live the inner experiences of running to their fullest. There is no program here, no routine. The exercises and visualizations are meant to be read, thought about, and, I hope, practiced. Experiment with them. Have fun with them. Approach them with an open mind. Don't expect anything to happen. Simply allow it to happen.

Standing Visualization

In some martial arts, aikido for example, students work to tap an awareness of self that lies just outside the skin. This source is often referred to as the energy body. (It corresponds to the feelings of good or poor vibes you might have around certain people.) Yogis in heightened states of awareness are said to have a force field that surrounds them. The simple awareness of your energy body can produce feelings of power for you while running. You can use a technique, borrowed from aikido black belt George Leonard, which enables two people to use their awareness of energy to transfer power.

Stand with your partner near a 100-yard interval section. Facing each other with palms facing a few inches apart and with one palm upward and one downward, let your eyes go "soft" and move your hands in a circular motion. Soon you will begin to feel sensations of warmth or electricity between your hands. Cultivate these sensations. Even if you have no feeling, pretend that it is there. Do this for a few minutes; then see how far away from each other's hands you can go while still feeling the connection. Note how close you have to remain to feel a bond.

Once this "charge" is built, your partner should drop his hands and face up the field. You, the "sending" partner, then transfer the energy that has been built up between you. You gather up the charge by bringing your own hands together as though you were holding a ball, and place the charge in the small of the back of your partner and send him on his way.

A good variation of this exercise is to have five or six people give energy to one. One person stands and the others place their hands a few inches away stroking the person's energy body. In my workshops this exercise has produced some very potent experiences. It is an excellent ritual before a hard workout or competition.

Restoring Energy

Visualization exercises can be used to restore energy during and after workouts. This practice has been studied carefully by the Soviets and East Germans. They call it psychic self-regulation and it is primarily known to us in the West through Dr. A. J. Lewis and the PSR Foundation in San Diego. The restoring process is a synthesis of Zen, yoga, Chinese medicine, autogenic training, and progressive relaxation. It is an exercise that will quicken recovery, return vitality, and relax strained postworkout muscles. It is usually most effective about two-thirds of the way through the workout, possibly just before the last set.

The exercise is best done standing. Find a comfortable place. If it is hot, get into the shade, cool down, put on your sweats. Your aim is to relax; you can do this with your imagination.

Start by imagining that you have lungs on the bottom of your feet so that each inhalation you take fills your body from the feet upward. Picture the breath you take as having a color—a color you identify with feeling refreshed. Take a number of easy, relaxing breaths and let the color fill your body and soothe you. Add a scent—again, one that you identify with refreshment. Now you may be breathing in yellow jasmine, green peppermint, or orange eucalyptus through the soles of your feet. Do this for five minutes and you will find that when you begin running again, you will feel refreshed.

This next visualization should be done on an open field during a fartlek workout. Its purpose is to develop calmness. With this visualization, no matter how vigorous physical activity becomes, you will be better able to maintain an inner quiet—a spot of unflappable imperturbability, the eye of a hurricane.

Begin by finding an area of the body in which you feel vitality and awareness. We'll experiment with three areas of the body: the abdomen, the chest, and the forehead.

Begin in the abdomen. Follow this into the upper chest and then into a place on the forehead between the eyes. Consciously bring breath to each of these vital centers. Then choose one of the areas to work with, the one in which you feel the most vitality or awareness. What we want to do is to create a point, spot, or place of stillness in the center of that area.

Begin with an in-breath and draw a line in your imagination around the outside of the chosen area. Let the line be solid but not too thick. Inhale a few more times, each time visualizing the lines of the circle. Now, on an exhalation, fill the circle completely up with black. Do this a number of times, making each circle smaller and smaller. On the inhalation you will be imagining a getting smaller circle with a line around it and on the exhalation you will fill the circle up. On each inhale and exhale you will make each circle smaller and smaller. On each exhale, as you fill the circle up, say the words "Relax," "Calm," and imagine the innermost point of the filled-in circle.

Continue the exercise until the exhaled black circle is only a dot, and the dot becomes synonymous with saying to yourself "Calm," "Relaxed." Begin running with soft eyes, imagining the dot or center of calmness. When the sense of the circle becomes unclear, stand and reprogram the breathing. In this way you will have established a natural fartlek. You should probably do simple gaits in this exercise so as to concentrate on the mental aspect.

Guided Fantasies

Here are some of the specific guided fantasies I spoke of in chapter IV.

1. Using Your Memories

The first guided fantasy has to do with looking into your past, in order to discover the situations behind the attitudes you have about your body, athletics, and physical activity.

Sit in a comfortable place, either in meditation position or lying on your back. Begin by taking a deep breath into your abdomen. Pick a spot just below the belly, and as you exhale imagine breathing air directly out your fingertips.

Now imagine a blank white billboard in your mind. Add a picture of a calendar with today's date.

Let the physical activity you have done or may do

today come into your mind. Imagine yourself *thoroughly enjoying* the activity. Imagine yourself feeling successful and pleased with the experience.

Next we are going to take a trip back into your past and think of the life we have lived up to this day. Think of time drifting, let the calendar fade and come again, just as if you were looking at a photograph. You have seen a calendar, you know what it looks like. Take the time period from the present back to 1970. Think of an event, a physical activity event representative of the time phase. This may be representative of your attitude toward your body at the time. Don't judge it, just watch it. Allow yourself to reexperience all aspects you can remember about this particular situation.

Now, do this same exercise for the following time periods: 1970–62, 1962–58, 1958–50, all the years back to the time just preceding your middle teens. If you're too young for long time periods, just go back two or three years at a time. In each time period let the memory of a physical activity represent the period and relive the memory in your mind.

Don't judge the memories. The purpose here is not to define some memories as "better" than others. If what honestly came up was a happy memory, relive it and relish it in a child's delight. If what you remember was a painful, anxious, maybe frustrating experience, let that surface also.

After a while, if your memory was happy, stay with it and make it even more happy. If the thought was sad, you have had that too long—let it drop. Replace it with the situation the way you would have liked it to have occurred. See, you've changed the script. See the same situation you felt bad about, and perform the activity successfully and happily. For a while, whatever your situation, let your mind remember a happy childhood physical activity.

Now let it all drop. Look at your mind again as the fair witness, observer of thoughts. After a while let yourself think of a positive memory from your teens or early twenties. Even if it is only walking through the woods on a beautiful fall day, or playing by yourself.

Whatever happy, successful, and positive memory comes to mind—let it occupy your thoughts. Notice what makes it feel the way it does. Are you relaxed? Did the image come easily? Was there something inexpressible? Did you like yourself? Next, let come to mind the memory of a physical activity or experience that is not quite what you would have liked it to have been. Maybe it was the time you struck out with the bases loaded when you were 13 years old. Or maybe it was a close basketball game your team lost. Relive the experience—it doesn't necessarily have to be a tragedy. Notice the context of the situation, the people you were with, the environment, what you and they were wearing. Look for a while, and then change this memory by making it the way you would have liked it to have occurred. Hit a home run. Sink the winning basket. After letting your mind watch itself again for a while, try to remember the most perfect physical activity day you have ever had. Look at all aspects of it—who you were with, why it felt so good.

If you can't remember a beautiful, perfect day, imagine what your perfect physical activity day would be like. Play the whole thing over again in your mind. Let yourself accept that you can get tremendous joy from your body. Play this story over and over in your mind and let this reality of happiness be a possibility for you.

When or just before it all gets fuzzy, begin breathing into the abdomen, and imagine yourself breathing out your fingertips. When the experience is completed for you, let your eyes open. Return to reality.

2. Body Sensations

This guided fantasy is best done just before going out for a workout, or perhaps before a race. It relates to a sense of body density—the sense of becoming light or heavy—and is akin to a martial arts demonstration in which, through self-suggestion, a person can become impossible to lift off the ground.

Start by standing still with your arms hanging by your sides. Imagine your arms extended *a mile* into the ground, and that at the end of the mile there are two clamps just made for your hands to slip under. Feel yourself very well grounded into the clamps.

Now imagine thick chocolate (yes, chocolate) coming down your body all the way to the waist. Feel it weighing you down and imagine yourself a solid, unmovable mountain. After you've been given these suggestions you should be all but impossible to lift. Try this giving the same instructions to someone.

Some people might describe what we're talking about here as self-hypnosis. Perhaps. Anyway, the purpose of it is to make you heavy. Why? Because ultimately we want to relax. So, in keeping with the doctrine of progressive relaxation we will first make ourselves heavy, then light. (In progressive relaxation techniques a muscle is tightened before it is allowed to relax.)

Here is the actual relaxing exercise. Lie on the floor with your arms extended, palms facing upward. Begin again by breathing into your belly and imagining that you are breathing out your fingertips.

Imagine that you have an opening or valve in the side of your neck. Each time you take a breath in, thick, heavy, but very clear oil begins filling the body. Let the oil enter the body. The first bit will sink to the places where your body makes contact with the floor. Let yourself feel the density of filling up. Then balloon outward so that you are more filled up than you can ever imagine. Be dense and unmovable as you lie on the ground. Stay with this sensation for a few moments.

Now imagine an outlet near your waist. Let the oily substance seep out slowly. As the heaviness leaves let the tension, pain, or fatigue you feel go with it. If you do this visualization properly you may feel almost devoid of physical presence. Think of yourself as the smallest possible particle that can lie on the ground.

To become light, begin breathing into the valve on the side of your neck again. This time, though, change the oxygen into imagined helium instead of oil, and with each breath feel lighter and lighter, as if your insides were like the insides of a bird. How beautiful it must feel for a bird to jump from one branch to another. With each breath feel the tingling of helium entering all the parts of your body from your toes to ankles, legs, abdomen, chest. After a while let your eyes open and take the feeling of lightness you are sensing into your actual work or workout.

3. Reality Perspective

The next guided fantasy is designed to give you a new perspective on reality. Begin again with breathing exercises that allow you to watch the flow of thoughts as they come through the mind. Practice the "fair witness" brand of meditation in which you separate out thoughts from the part of yourself that watches the thoughts. Now imagine that your thoughts are occurring, not in your mind, but in an area as large as the room you are sitting in.

Think of where you are standing. Suppose it's New York City, the island of Manhattan. Now expand your mind by thinking thoughts which you may have had before, but which you don't contemplate too often. Imagine your mind hovering above the island of Manhattan, looking down upon it. Notice the tall buildings, perhaps Central Park. Your mind is above these things looking down upon them. Give your mind the power to accomplish this.

Next, let your mind hover over the whole state of New York; notice the contours of the roads, the changes in the land, the trail of highways. Let your mind expand out even farther so that you are looking at the whole of the United States, and then the United States as if you were in a spaceship looking down on the earth. Let the image just come and as it does, look down on the entire planet. Notice the globular sphere, the various continents, the way the water bodies connect with the land masses. Your mind is outside, hovering on the edge of the universe. On one side, circling around the earth, is the moon. From that image, look toward the sun, but not directly. (The rays might harm your eyes!) Nearer to the sun are the planets Mercury and Venus. Farther away are Mars and our largest planet, Jupiter; then a planet with a large ring around it, Saturn.

Now your mind, your awareness is way out in the solar system. You are feeling very expansive, perhaps even cosmic. Look as far out in the solar system as possible, and see the farthest planets: Uranus, Neptune, and Pluto. Look back at the solar system from this perspective. Feel the wonderful quiet; the sounds of meteors whizzing past. You have never felt so excited and yet so peaceful. Looking back, you realize that the solar system is finite, but it is ever expanding, and there is no edge—space goes farther and farther out.

Earth is part of a solar system that is infinite, ever expanding, and has no edge. With this idea in mind, watch your mind for a while. See if the trip we have been on has changed the natural flow of thoughts going through your mind. Now think about the body that is attached to your head and mind. Your body is made up of atoms and molecules that have an identity. From a different perspective, the molecules in your body are the same as molecules in a chair or wall. They don't stick together. So you, the runner who goes down the street, are part of the ordinary commerce of life, which exists in a universe, in a solar system that is infinite, ever expanding, and without an edge. There is no way out of this situation. Think about this for a while.

Now come back into the room. Your mind can close down a bit. Instead of the whole solar system, just dwell on the earth, and perhaps Mercury, Venus, and Mars. Then focus down on just the earth, then the United States, the East, New York State, and finally the island of Manhattan. Let the thoughts in your mind occur in a space as large as the room in which you are sitting. Then for a while watch your own thoughts, and finally open your eyes.

Body Image Meditation

The body image guided fantasy begins by taking a close look at your physical self and the image you have of yourself. The end of the guided fantasy will have you visualizing a physical activity performed perfectly. The fantasy goes something like this:

Close your eyes. Relax by taking a breath into your abdomen and visualizing that you are breathing out your fingertips. Let your first mental picture be the image of yourself walking out into a large grassy meadow. Notice how soft and fragrant the environment is. You can hear the sounds of birds chirping. You are secure and lighthearted. There is a large rock on the meadow. Begin walking toward the rock. It's a large rock but easy to climb.

You are on top of the rock, sitting in a comfortable position that looks out toward the horizon. As you look out, you notice that across the meadow is a body of water with a ship moored at a dock. Don't hurry; let yourself just relax, feeling secure and happy. After a while a transparent cloudlike covering surrounds you. You are sitting inside it—as if inside a protective cocoon. You have a small light inside the cloud for looking at places you can't see directly with your eyes.

Begin with the feet. Think, first, of the bottom of your feet. In your mind's eye, visualize how your arch is shaped. Notice the shape of your toes; then place your awareness around your Achilles tendon. What, if any place, on your foot is sore? Do you generally feel confidence in your feet? Now let's move up the leg. Remember, you can use the light inside the cloud to scan any section of your body you cannot see directly with your eyes. Focus your attention on your calf muscle. Trace the calf from your Achilles to behind your knee. What is your calf shaped like? Next, the shin. Has it ever been sore? Move up to the knees. Look all around and through your knees. Notice how they are designed, the places of bone and the conclaves mixing tendons, ligaments, and muscle. Is any part of your knee sore? Can you pinpoint the spot? Are there any peculiar crackings or sounds when your knees move? Let your awareness go up and down the front and back of the legs observing for soreness and/or tightness and pain.

Now move farther up the leg. Imagine your thighs

and hamstrings. Picture in your mind what your thighs and hamstrings are shaped like. Do you carry excess weight in that part of your body? Is there soreness or tightness in your upper legs? Now probe your lower back and pinpoint places of soreness or pain. Do you tighten your buttocks muscles? Look throughout your lower back; try to get a sense of the flowing of sinew into bones. Do you notice any strain in this part of your body, any tightness or lack of confidence?

Bring your awareness to the front of the body. Place it near the diaphragm and around the abdomen. Can you feel extra weight in and around your center? What about the sides of your body, just above the waist? The Chinese say the best place to focus attention is just below the belly. Here, in the Chinese view, is the body's source of movement when it is "centered." Breathe into this place. How often do you have a sense of moving from this location in your body?

Dwell on the way you feel about your whole lower body. Scan the whole area, noting places of soreness and tension. Move up to the chest, the lungs. Breathe in gently through the hair in your nostrils. Let the air fill your entire lung area. Gently note the sensibilities of your lungs. Do you feel confidence in your lungs' ability to provide oxygen on demand? Feel the dimensions and limits of your lungs. Would you say you have confidence in your lungs?

Sense the space between your neck and shoulders. Is there tightness there? Do your shoulders rise up to the ears in moments of fear? Starting from your lower back, trace your spinal cord all the way up to your neck. Can you notice places of soreness, special sections of rigidity? Would you say you have a supple or a stiff spine? What about the fleshy part next to the spine on the upper back?

Mentally look down your forearms, and into your hands. Do you feel expressive or artistic? Place your awareness on your facial area. Sense the expression in the eyes, the set of the chin, the tension or lack of it in the brow. What of your eyes, your cheeks? Go to the top of your head, your hair, the back of your neck. Relax now and take a long look at your whole body. Notice individual parts, notice too how you feel overall. Sense your identity: your body and personality. How do you feel about your body and yourself? Rest with it all for a while.

Now go through your entire body again. This time, instead of taking the body as it is, change it into your idealized self. Visualizing how you want to change your body can move your body in that direction. Imagine the outcome of a desire, and the mind often works out the path for achievement.

Begin with the feet. Place your awareness in your feet. Make them strong and free from soreness. Place awareness in your calves. Shape them as you want them; give them strength and flexibility. Let your shins be free from soreness. Let the knee move acording to its function.

Imagine your lower back without soreness. Imagine that the center of yourself is just below your belly and you are walking with calmness and certainty. Let your entire spine be fluid and flexible. Give your upper back strength. Let your lungs be bellowslike. Feel the air coming through the nostrils, endowing your lungs with great power and endurance. Let your upper arms have strength without muscle bulk. Picture your hands as beautiful, expressive, artistic. Eliminate tension between shoulders and neck. Place your awareness in your facial area and imagine what it would be like if you had done years of spiritual seeking. Give your face the look of a found seeker after years of search. Place your awareness on your hair. See if you can locate one strand of hair.

Remember, you are doing this sitting on top of a rock that overlooks a beautiful meadow. There is a large body of water in the distance. It is midday. The sun comes out and begins to burn off the cloudlike covering. The tanning rays of the sun, the smell of the grass, and the distant ocean mist relax you. You feel as powerful and playful as you have ever felt in your life. Sit there for a moment, feeling your "new" self and taking in the powerful rays of the sun. You are tanned, in a good mood, possessing your perfect body. The story now accelerates. Allow yourself to step off the rock and onto the meadow. You will soon imagine yourself performing a physical activity as perfectly as you have ever imagined, with your body doing all the beautiful and aesthetically powerful and graceful actions of a long-to-be-remembered peak of mind/body experience.

Now let it happen. Allow yourself to experience a physical activity. Although the experience is only in your mind, if the imagination is vibrant enough it will almost be like accomplishing the acts. Let the imagined experience begin. See yourself in the early stages of an activity, feeling vibrant, sensing kinesthetic beauty and aesthetic delight. Go to the midpoint of the experience. Pinpoint the concentration there, with your body still moving in the fantasy, expressing its full potential. Finally, enter the climactic time of the experience. Feel dominant, powerful. Experience a far-reaching confidence and happiness. Let yourself end the experience successfully, doing better than ever before and realizing all that you didn't while you were in a relaxed playful concentrative mood.

Stay with this experience as long as it gives you a clear picture. As the image begins to fade, let yourself walk toward the water. Feel the wonderful sense of having experienced something that you will remember for a long time. It will stay just below your conscious level, as a special way of knowing.

You reach the mooring. There is a large ship there with the gangplank thrown down. On the ship are all your friends and relatives. They notice your changes, they realize what you have just experienced. You are pleased, relaxed, and inexhaustibly happy. When the ship has gone out to sea in another place and time zone you begin to return to the person who first entered the meadow. You are going to remember this memory—this process toward your own truth. This memory will return to you from an unconscious place when the situation of the right magnitude appears.

To come out of this, begin breathing into your abdomen and imagine letting the air out of your fingertips.

When your eyes open you will be satisfied and happy. You will have a sense of deep fulfillment.

Mental Rehearsal Before Race or Workout

The following exercise is best done before a difficult workout. Its purpose is to help you develop an attitude of success toward a race or hard workout. Research in mental visualization shows that when you couple physical practice with visualizing, you enhance your chances of a successful performance.

Start this exercise by finding a quiet place to sit or lie in. As soon as you're comfortable, imagine yourself at the site of the race or workout. Notice the clothes that you are wearing, and imagine yourself as happy, relaxed, and confident. As if you are playing a movie to yourself, watch yourself beginning your performance. Begin with the early parts of the race. See yourself running in the early parts of the race with power, ease, and confidence. Notice that you are relaxed and that everything seems to be going according to plan. Your body is loose, there is no tension or pain anywhere. Visualize yourself going past the midpoint of the race, still running strongly. Follow this with the climactic stage. Notice that you have gotten through the time-space in which it could have been difficult. You hung on and it is going well. You experience a boost of energy, a second wind. In your mind's eye you finish feeling stronger, more vital, successful, and dominating than you have in a long time.

Play this like a movie in your mind. Do it for days and weeks before a major contest. Picturing yourself successful, relaxed, and on top of things will further your success and pleasure in racing.

The Running Sesshin

The purpose of this exercise is to integrate mind and body while you run, to help you observe the contents of your mind while you are moving. You can achieve a great deal through this exercise: lessening of the anxiety of getting the run over with, for one, plus the ability to know what you are thinking. When you achieve presence in the actual moment, you more fully experience your run.

"Sesshin" is a term taken from Zen training. In some Zen practice, certain periods are set aside for sitting meditation, interspersed with walking meditation. A sesshin may last a day, or even longer. Eating and sleeping become part of the experience. In my workshop sesshin we combine a running section with the walking. Usually there are three sets: sitting, walking, and running. The three sets can last from 40 minutes to an hour. At least two sets of 20 minutes each are necessary to feel the benefit of the exercise. For a narrative of a running sesshin that was done with Michael Murphy, I refer you to the story "Running into the Spirit" in my book *Running Home.*

You begin this Zen practice by closing your eyes and observing the natural flow of your breath. Follow the breath, counting each inhalation and exhalation up to the count of four: "One" on the inhale, "Two" on the exhale, "Three" on the inhale, "Four" on the exhale. Continue this for about five minutes of the first meditation session, which should last at least ten minutes. The counting enables you to slow the mind down. Spend another few minutes just counting on the exhale up to four. The last few minutes, free yourself from the observation of breaths and watch your thoughts from a position of detached awareness. This means to observe your thoughts without judgment. You may be thinking of the chore you forgot to do, last week's laundry, a fight you had with your neighbor. Whatever, just observe without judgment.

Then move into a walk. As you get up from your sitting position, use the "soft eyes" technique. This will enable you to watch your mind, or create a mental picture in your mind while still having enough vision to run. Let your eyes be half-closed in an unstressful half squint. Standing from the seated position, place your left hand in a fist and cover it with the right hand. Begin a slow walk. This walk, referred to as the Zen walk, is not meant to get you anywhere. Its purpose is to take the sitting meditation consciousness into movement, into action. The step is slow. Touching first your heel, then rolling onto the toes, and finally swinging the opposite leg to the front and again hitting heel and rolling to toes. So it is, heel, toes, swing, and so on. The walk should produce a settling effect. At first you may feel off balance, but after a while you should come to enjoy the concentrated dynamic you are building up for the run. Your aim should be to keep some part of your body in motion at all times, even if it is an imperceptible motion. Your walk should be done either in a circle or in a straight line that leads to the running surface. It should last about a third of the sitting session, about three or four minutes.

We are now almost ready to run. At our workshops, the group at this point is instructed to stand still, with hands dropped by the sides. Everyone's gaze is downward, the idea being to focus attention inward. You pick out a blade of grass, a crevice in the cement, whatever is near you that comes to your attention. Once you start running, should you begin to lose your awareness, you simply stop and focus on a spot while watching your thoughts. Use this time to regain awareness of your consciousness and/or as a necessary rest period.

We then run in a circle. It works best if the circle is no smaller than 300 yards around but no larger than a half mile. The idea is to take the last part of the sitting meditation, watching thoughts, and carry it into the running. While running, keep paying attention to the stream of thoughts that come through the mind. Remember, anytime you become physically tired or lose connection with awareness you can stop, stand still, and return to the standing focusing.

What usually occurs in a group session is that a circle forms which has no beginning or end. Some people are stopped, others are joining in. The circle becomes a group running without a leader or front or back. Usually you run at a shuffle or fresh swing tempo. Each individual has an option because no one is competing. After leading the first lap I stand in the middle of the circle and direct the group while watching and occasionally making comments. I will stop the group at an appropriate point, and have them wait in meditation until the rest of the group assembles. We then return to the meditation circle.

With each successive meditation I try to take the awareness deeper. Then begin by counting just on the exhale to four, but quickly move to counting inhale and exhale up to ten. And when a person loses count of the breaths, return to the count of one on the inhale. (Done correctly you won't get to ten too often.) The walking and standing is repeated, and the running in a circle with the option of stopping. Usually I take ten minutes for the meditation, three or four minutes for the walking, a minute or so for the standing, and seven to ten minutes for the running. I sometimes say things to people as they pass, either for an individual to flow in with the group, or to drop the thought I feel they are carrying in their minds. It can be like the Zen teacher who hits the dozing meditator with a bamboo stick. In the third set the observation of breath is only on the exhale up to ten and there is at least half the time for observation of thoughts. After this exercise some people report that, for the first time, they aren't anxious while running. Some feel as if they are not running at all, and some say that they have never before had an awareness of what went on in their minds while they were running.

You can do this in place of one of your long runs or as a fartlek workout. The whole process may take longer than you usually spend, but this is the nature of a sesshin anyway. Even if you do this once a month you will benefit from a physical and spiritual vantage.

Autogenic Recovery After Workouts

This is best done after the running workout to promote recovery and relaxation. Begin by making yourself comfortable and warm. Put on your sweats and lie on your back. Take some deep breaths into your abdomen. I am going to give you some suggestions, and when I do you will repeat them silently to yourself. Focus your awareness in your arms, and say to yourself, "My arms are very heavy. My arms are very heavy." Repeat this to yourself five or six times. Follow this with the inner silent statement, "I feel completely relaxed and calm." The statement "I am relaxed and calm" will follow every suggestion exercise. Repeat to yourself silently five or six times, "My legs are very heavy, my legs are very heavy," then "I feel relaxed and calm. I feel completely relaxed and calm."

Let a light flow of air come through the nostrils. Let it completely fill the lungs and abdomen. Say silently to yourself, "My lungs are cool and relaxed, my lungs are cool and relaxed." Then repeat again, "I am relaxed and calm. I am completely relaxed and calm."

Next place your awareness in your abdomen area. Say silently to yourself, "I feel warm and flowing in my abdomen. I feel warm and flowing in my abdomen." Repeat this five or six times followed by the statement "I am relaxed and calm. I am completely relaxed and calm."

Finally say to yourself, "My forehead is very cool, my forehead is very cool." Repeat this to yourself five or six times, followed by saying silently "I am relaxed and calm. I am completely relaxed and calm." Finally, lie for a few moments breathing into your abdomen, and imagining yourself breathing out your fingertips. Do this until you are ready to allow your eyes to open.

V

Breathing and Stretching

It's hard for me to think of two aspects that are more central to the running experience and yet more neglected (even by coaches) than breathing and stretching. If you work on nothing else for the next two weeks but breathing and stretching, I can guarantee that your running will improve. You'll run more smoothly, more powerfully, and more enjoyably.

The idea behind developing your breathing powers is to forestall the anaerobic state when you run. Contrary to what many people think, the point at which you switch from aerobic running to anaerobic running isn't fixed. By breathing properly, you can postpone the onset of anaerobia longer than someone who may have the same maximum oxygen consumption level as you but uses it less efficiently. As for stretching—well, it's an accepted principle of running training (finally) that the best way to avoid the most common running injuries is to do a regular series of stretching exercises to compensate for the impact that running has on the muscles that get the most workout during a run.

Breathing Basics

Everybody knows how to breathe—it's an instinct we're born with—but not everybody knows how to breathe properly. Relatively few runners know how to breathe in a way that enables them to get the most out of their oxygen delivery system.

Proper breathing is not stylized breathing. The Finnish breathing system, for example, in which you try to take two breaths in every two steps, works OK for a relaxing run but it doesn't work under stress. Even when exertion becomes moderate, the Finnish technique is inoperable. No, the only way to achieve greater lung power is by doing exercises that develop proper breathing techniques.

Breathing Exercises

The exercises developed by master running coach Percy Cerutty (full lung aeration) and the man referred to as "Dr. Breathe," Carl Stough (breathing coordination), seem to me to be the best place to begin. Both men teach breathing techniques that strengthen the involuntary muscles and correct inefficient breathing patterns, and we'll be borrowing techniques from both.

The Exhale

Most people are under the impression that the important part of the breathing cycle is the breath you take in. The opposite is true—especially when it comes to breathing while you run. The biggest problem runners who don't breathe properly face is that *they don't get rid of enough stale air when they breathe out.* The stale air literally sticks to their lungs. The point of the exhale isn't merely to empty out enough air so that you can breathe in again. It's to get rid of *all* the air containing waste products so that the incoming air isn't contaminated and you benefit from the full measure of its oxygen content.

How do you know when you've cleaned your

lungs of stale air? It's not easy to answer. Cerutty and Stough insist that noise—natural noise—is the only dependable way of knowing for certain. "The noise," explains Cerutty, "confirms the expelling of air."

Try it yourself. Take a deep breath and then breathe out naturally, as you normally do. Breathe in again, trying to get a feel for how much air you're taking in. Then exhale again, but this time do it making a sharp "hu" sound, and take note of how much air you're able to take in when you breathe in the next time.

The Inhale

Most people don't know how to breathe out or in properly. The center of your breathing mechanism is in the middle of your body—the diaphragm—but this doesn't mean that you breathe "through your stomach."

Think of it this way. Your lungs have a primary and secondary tank. The primary tank is the diaphragm; the secondary tank is the chest. As Stough explains, "The lungs should be filled with air from the bottom to the top, just as a container is filled."

In order to breathe from bottom to top you need a strong supporting abdomen. The easiest way to check the strength of your abdomen is by observing how your body responds to the locust pose in the stretching set. If you have difficulty doing these stretching exercises, chances are your abdomen needs more work.

As for inhaling, don't be afraid to breathe through both nose and mouth. Only by using both can you get maximum inhalation. And when you breathe in, don't hesitate to use your shoulders. One of the first things Cerutty taught me was to actually say the word "Shoulders" when I breathed in so that I would remember to lift my shoulders and allow the air's atmospheric pressure to fill my diaphragm and lungs.

Breathing Exercises

Each of the exercises described below was developed by Stough, Cerutty, or a world-class runner. They are all very useful in improving your breathing.

1. Supine Breathing

Carl Stough, who has also worked with the Yale track team, used this exercise to help Americans prepare for the high-altitude Olympics at Mexico City (1968). The 6800-foot altitude posed a double problem for the Olympians: performance and recovery. The point of this exercise was to help the Americans regulate their breathing cycle so that they could run with more power and rhythm and recover with less trouble.

Start by lying on your back. On your exhale, count out loud to 10, keeping the exhale relaxed until the end of the audible count. Breathe in normally and on the next exhale, increase the number of your audible count to 15.

Repeat the process, extending the count by fives on each exhale. You will notice that as your exhale increases, your inhale will increase. If the lower abdomen begins to tense or if you're forcing, stop counting

This is as much a relaxation exercise as it is a breath control exercise, so don't force it. Generally, if you're in reasonable shape, you should be able to count to a hundred for each 20 seconds of exhale, but after your breathing muscles have developed a little bit, you may be able to extend to 30 or 40 seconds on a single breath. Stough recommends this exercise as a daily practice and as a prerace relaxation exercise.

2. Breathing and Walking

This exercise was developed by Cerutty, who recommends it as a means of practicing emptying and filling of the lungs while you walk.

As you walk, you fill the lungs to their fullest capacity. (If done correctly, this will take you about five to eight paces, and in the process you will probably draw yourself to full height.)

Expel the air forcefully, concentrating on getting rid of every last bit of air in the lungs. To do this you will probably have to lean over until the upper part of your trunk is almost parallel with the ground.

(If you're self-conscious, you probably won't want to do this while you're walking in public, but it's a good exercise to practice when you are home alone, or walking by yourself.)

3. Stationary Breath Holding

This little exercise was a favorite of the Czech running great Emil Zatopek, who used to practice it while walking in the woods, as a means of developing his willpower.

Start by counting the number of steps you can take holding one breath. Once you've recovered your breath, try it again, with the idea of increasing the number of steps.

4. Blowing Out the Candle

This is a technique for cleansing your lungs of carbon dioxide and allowing fresh oxygen to flow in. It's best done after an anaerobic run. All you do while walking slowly is exhale forcefully, as if you were blowing out the candles on a cake.

5. Tidal Breathing

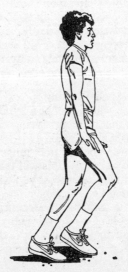

Tidal breathing—exhale

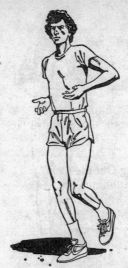

Tidal breathing—inhale into diaphragm

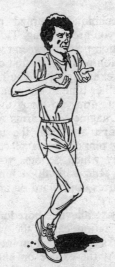

Tidal breathing—inhale into lungs

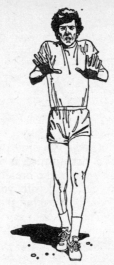

Tidal breathing—exhale of tidal breath

This is a technique I learned from Percy Cerutty. You do it while you are running. Tidal breathing is best done at the junction point between two gaits. As you approach the junction point, your first objective is to empty your lungs by exhaling. Now you have access to more air than at any other time in the breathing cycle. On the inhale, bring your arms up along the sides with palms facing inward. Imagine your arms as an elevator. Fill the diaphragm first and then the upper lobes of the lungs. Finish by pinpointing a place in the middle of your chest cavity which denotes you have completely filled the lungs. Run with filled lungs for a moment, then throw the arms downward on an exhale and accelerate into a faster gait.

A good way to alleviate boredom during the run is to add a visualization called the wave to your tidal breath. This works best during an interval. Start the run with soft eyes. At the exhale on entering the junction point, imagine a wave gathering. On the inhale picture the wave rising, and on the final exhale let the wave crest and ride it to the shore.

6. Shoulder Breathing

Shoulder breathing is a variation of tidal breathing. It helps your endurance by relaxing your body and by bringing you back to yourself; that is, becoming "centered."

Shoulder breathing resembles a shrug. While you run, empty all the air from your lungs. Then lift your shoulders. This lift will create more space and atmospheric pressure in the lungs. As you exhale, propel your body forward. A good visualization is to imagine yourself already at the spot where the breathing ends. Then, on the exhale, try to catch up with yourself. Shoulder breathing is a good way of breaking the monotony of a long continuous run.

Naturalistic running movements use the same respiration principle. In cantering or galloping, for instance, the lead arm is thrown forward with an exhale

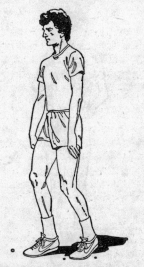

Shoulder breathing—exhale

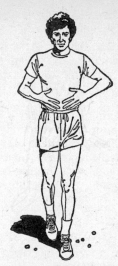

Shoulder breathing—inhale into diaphragm

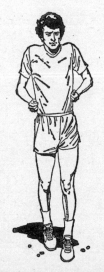

Shoulder breathing—lift shoulders for full breath

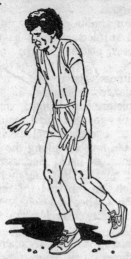

Shoulder breathing—exhale of shoulder breath

synchronized with a bounding off the opposite foot. This
thrusts the body into a longer stride. When this step is
integrated into the other strides the run becomes asymmetrical, the canter step being longer than the others,
which are of shorter and equal length.

Stretching

Stretching has only recently become an accepted
part of the distance runner's training regimen. The
reason is that stretching and other calisthenics don't
produce much in the way of cardiovascular benefit.
What's more, track coaches have long been in disagree-
ment over the value of flexibility. Arthur Lydiard,
for example, recommended only some limited leg
swings and tendon stretching. Cerutty suggested sit-ups
and hanging from parallel bars and gymnastic appara-
tus, but no more. And if you were one of Igloi's runners,
you needed special permission to stretch. Igloi believed

changing gaits and a grass running surface were all you needed to keep loose.

So except for traditional stretching exercises used by sprinters and hurdlers, runners have long neglected stretching exercises, just as Eastern yogis, whose chief form of exercise is stretching, have long neglected cardiovascular fitness. The result: unfit yogis and sore, muscularly unbalanced runners.

Happily, the picture has changed, and none too soon. For as exercise physiologists now realize, running produces a state of overdevelopment in the so-called prime movers—the muscles along the back of the leg, the thigh, and the low back. Because of this overdevelopment, these muscles become short and inflexible, causing the muscles in the front of the leg, the thigh, and the abdomen to become relatively weak. Hence the need for flexibility exercises to correct the imbalance.

Another reason for flexibility exercises is to counteract the punishment that your muscles take during a run.

As Robert Anderson, who has made a career out of suggesting stretching routines for runners, says:

> On any given run, the runner experiences, to some degree, microscopic tears of the musculators. These tiny tears lead to the formation of scar tissue (scar tissue does not have the properties to stretch) and to increased muscle inflexibility and stiffness. This is a very injury prone condition and unless the negative effects of running can be minimized and brought under control by proper and regular stretching, the runner has a good chance of being injured.

The flexibility exercises that appear in this chapter were developed by Dr. Kenneth Dychtwald, author of *Bodymind*. Dr. Dychtwald insists that much of the pain and the soreness that runners experience can be minimized through a regular program of flexibility exercises, and I couldn't agree more. I have selected

these particular exercises because they are designed
to free up all the joints in the body, increase flexibility
in the back of the body, and in the process improve
neuromuscular function. What's more, this particular
exercise set provides a comfortable balance of forward and backward bending poses, as well as a blend
of twisting, rotating, arching, and inverting positions.

The overall aim is to develop flexibility throughout the whole body, not just basic running muscles.
Our concern in this program is to do more than keep
the legs from cramping. We are working toward op-
timizing total health and well-being.

There are three variations on this set. The short
routine (exercises designated by an asterisk), or the
full 17 exercises should be done before you run. The
four exercises designated by a double asterisk should
be done after your run. A full set takes about 30
minutes (including appropriate rest periods); a half set,
20 minutes. The afterward exercises take 5 minutes.

If you are unable to achieve a completed position,
simply move into the posture as far as you comfortably
can and stop when you feel a mild strain. The point
of strain marks one of the many "edges" that exist
within your body and identifies a point of limited flexibility. *Do not try to force yourself past this edge.*
Instead, as Bob Anderson suggests, "Sometimes it is
a good idea to do stretches with your eyes closed to
help feel the stretch more and for greater relaxation."

Whatever your level, if you perform these exercises correctly, sensitively, and regularly, they will help
you become supple and more graceful. Not only will
they facilitate and enhance your running development, they will bring you to a feeling of pleasure and
satisfaction.

Some General Tips

1. When to Exercise

The best time of day is in the morning before
breakfast, in the late afternoon before dinner, or at

least 90 minutes after eating. These stretches should
be practiced at least once daily, right before running
if you're a serious runner.

2. Where to Exercise

A roomy, well-ventilated area where physical and
psychological distractions are at a minimum is the best
place to exercise. These exercises require a flat surface, and you'll need space to stretch your trunk and
limbs without interference. If possible, always practice in the same "exercise sanctuary," so that your
exercise space will become a special place in your
daily life—a place where you can comfortably retreat
and focus on yourself. If you intend to practice these
stretches outdoors, select a comfortable, level environment where you can pay close attention to yourself and not be distracted by noise or people.

3. Ground Cover

Cover your practice surface with a large towel,
mat, or pad. Choose the covering carefully and be
sure that you will feel comfortable using it with your
exercises. Put it away when it is not in use. If you
practice these exercises inside as well as outside, use
two mats.

4. Clothing

When you exercise, wear comfortable, loose-fitting
clothing—as little as possible. The less clothing you
wear, the more chance your skin has to breathe. Clothing should never bind or restrict you. Remove eye-
glasses, watches, and any confining jewelry. (You may
wish to keep a clock or watch handy to time certain
exercises.) Always remove your running shoes.

5. Rhythm

It is best to perform all the stretches every day
when you exercise. If your time is limited, do not
rush through the exercises, but choose six or seven that
you feel are most helpful. You are better off doing
6 stretches correctly than 12 incorrectly. Your body

responds as much to your attitude while exercising as to the specific exercises.

6. Awareness
If you take your time and concentrate on these exercises, they will help give you a better understanding and more sensitive appreciation of your unique body and mind. The exercises are not overly difficult or demanding. If you are in good health, you should be able to take each position to within 75 percent of completion. As you perform the stretches, note which ones are easier or harder for you and, correspondingly, which parts of your body need the least or most work.

7. Attitude
Think of your exercise practice as a time of pleasure and adventure, rather than a rigid discipline or self-punishment. If you feel like skipping a session or two, skip it and forget it. Allow yourself to enjoy these exercises and you will find yourself looking forward to your next session.

Stretches

1. Standing Full-Body Swing*
Technique: Stand comfortably erect with your feet at shoulder width apart. Inhale and slowly raise your arms. Extend them out to either side, parallel to the floor, palms down. Slowly swing your body all the way to your right side (your entire body, from ankles to neck). When you've swung as far to the right as is comfortably possible, reverse directions and swing all the way around to the left. Breathe deeply and relax your entire body as you perform these swings. Continue swinging back and forth for a count of 20. Then exhale and slowly lower your arms back to your side.

Benefit: This is an excellent warm-up for loosening muscles and joints before running. It energizes nerves and muscles of the spine and is helpful for trimming the waist and stretching the muscle in the front, back, and sides of legs.

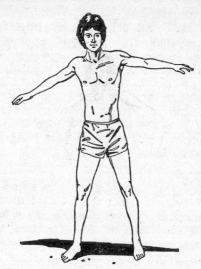

Standing full body swing

2. Pelvic Rotation

Technique: Stand comfortably erect with your feet at shoulder width apart. Relax your body and place your hands on your hips. Breathe deeply and slowly and as you do move your hips around in a wide circular motion. Try not to lead with your shoulders or head. Instead, allow your pelvis to initiate all of the movements. Breathe deeply. Try to move your hips in the widest possible circles until you have performed this exercise ten times. Then relax for a few moments and perform the exercise ten times in the opposite direction.

Variation: Try this exercise with your knees bent slightly. Doing so will lower your center of gravity several inches, and will shift some of the focus of the movement to the muscles of your thighs and calves and free up your pelvis—all this while strengthening your legs.

Benefits: This exercise will help bring a measure of grace and ease to all motion and activity, especially running. It will free up the muscle that surrounds the pelvis area and connect it to the legs below and the spine above. It will also tone the muscle sheaths

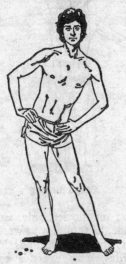

Pelvic rotation

that wrap around the front, back, and sides of the body and stimulate circulation and neuromuscular coordination. Finally, it will keep your lower back supple and help your legs and hips remain free-moving and flexible.

3. Grape Picking*

Technique: Stand comfortably erect with your feet at shoulder width apart. Inhale deeply as you slowly stretch both arms high overhead. Breathing deeply, stretch your right hand as high as possible, simultaneously pushing your heels downward, the better to fully extend the entire right side of your body. Breath-

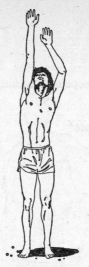

Grape picking

ing deeply, repeat on the left side. Continue reaching upward side to side, as though you were picking grapes. Repeat ten times, then exhale and slowly lower your arms to your sides. This exercise can also be performed while standing on your toes instead of pushing downward with your heels, to further strengthen and vitalize your feet, ankles, and calves.

Variation 1: While lying on your back, allow your entire body to relax and, with your arms extended back over your head, alternate stretching the right and left sides of your body. Be sure to stretch fully, creating the greatest distance between the fingertips and heels.

Variation 2: When you extend your right hand away from your body, relax your right leg and extend your left leg. Then stretch your left arm and right leg. The force of the stretch will crisscross your body, thereby further toning the related musculature.

Benefits: This is a full-body stretch that not only relieves everyday fatigue and tension but restores energy and suppleness to the entire body. It elasticizes all the muscles in the back of the legs that you use when you run, and it lengthens major muscles of the torso and limbs. Additionally, this exercise gently expands the chest and stretches the diaphragm and abdomen, which deepens breathing and improves circulation.

4. Triangle Pose*

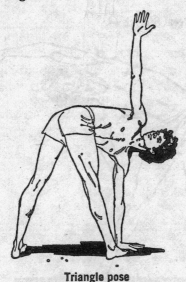

Triangle pose

Technique: Stand comfortably erect with your legs two to three feet apart. Inhale and slowly raise your arms and extend them out to either side, parallel to the floor, palms down. Exhale and slowly twist your body to the right, simultaneously reaching toward your right foot with your left hand. As you do this, keep your right arm relaxed and extended upward and turn your head to look toward it. Breathe deeply and hold this position for a count of ten. Then inhale deeply as you return to a standing position.

First extend your arms outward and then lower them to your sides. Relax and repeat to the other side.

Benefits: The triangle pose helps keeps leg muscles flexible and stress-free. It tones and vitalizes the muscles and nerves of the spine, gently massages muscle and viscera of the abdominal region, and aids digestion and elimination. It also helps trim the waist, and strengthens and elasticizes the lower back and buttocks.

5. Lateral Stretch

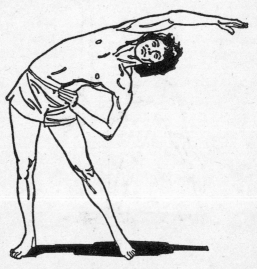

Lateral stretch

Technique: Stand comfortably erect, feet parallel and at shoulder width apart. Slowly raise your right arm straight overhead, simultaneously placing your left hand on your left hip. Inhale deeply, then exhale, allowing your body to bend as far as possible to the left while reaching over and down to the left with your right arm. As you hold this posture you should breathe deeply, your head and face forward. Resist the tendency to twist or bend your body either forward or backward. Hold for a count of ten and then slowly return to an upright position. Relax and reverse sides.

The lateral stretch elasticizes the muscles on the inside and outside of the legs, reducing unnecessary stiffness for runners. It lengthens many of the lateral muscles of the body that are important in all movement, yet seldom exercised. It also frees muscle tension surrounding the pelvis and lower back, aids in trimming the waist, and tones joints, tendons, and ligaments.

6. Wall Stretch*

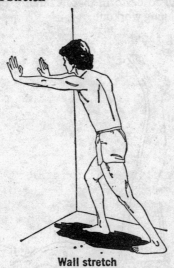

Wall stretch

Technique: Stand comfortably with your feet at shoulder width apart about an arm's length from a sturdy wall or tree. Raise your arms and place your hands firmly on the wall with your fingers pointing upward. Then move your left foot back 1 or 2 feet behind the other and place it heel down, toes straight ahead. Lean into the wall and allow all of the muscles, tendons, and ligaments of your left leg to stretch and lengthen. Breathe deeply and hold for a count of ten. Return to the neutral standing position and relax. Repeat this exercise with the other leg.

Variation: As you position your legs for this wall stretch, bend your knees slightly so as to deepen the stretch. Hold for a count of ten and repeat with the other leg.

Benefits: This stretch is especially important to runners because it acts specifically to stretch and lengthen the muscles, tendons, and ligaments in the back of the legs and lower back that are usually tightened and thickened during all running activity. It is particularly helpful to perform these exercises before and after each running workout.

7. Leg Lifts*

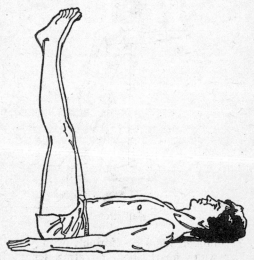

Leg lift—raise both legs off the floor

Technique: Lie flat on your back with your arms to your sides. Breathe deeply and allow your entire body to relax. Inhale and slowly raise both of your legs off of the floor and elevate them as high as you are comfortably able. Keeping your legs relaxed and straight, breathe normally and hold this position for a count of ten. Then slowly exhale while allowing your legs to gradually return to the floor. Perform twice.

Variation: Lie on your back and relax your entire body. Inhale deeply and slowly lift your left leg and el-

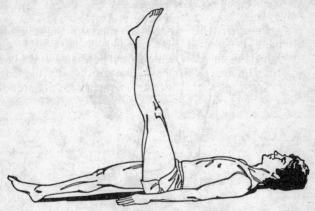

Leg lift—raise your left leg

evate it as high as you are able. Keeping your leg straight and relaxed, breathe normally and hold this position for a count of ten. Then slowly exhale while allowing your legs to gradually return to the floor.

Benefits: Leg lifts strengthen back and abdominal muscles while stretching many of the muscles in the lower back and legs. Especially good for runners because it stimulates and tones the abdominal viscera and keeps the lower back, hip, and groin stress-free. The single leg lifts are additionally helpful because they encourage more integrated and flexible connections between each leg and the spine.

8. Standing Forward Bend (Hands to Feet)

Technique: Stand comfortably erect with your feet shoulder width apart. Raise your arms high overhead as you inhale deeply. Then exhale slowly and bend your body forward so that your hands touch your toes and your nose moves toward your knees. Your knees should not be bent or locked, as either of these devia-

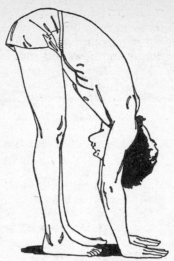

Standing forward bend

tions would shift the focus of the stretch away from the muscles that could benefit from the gentle strain of this posture. Hold the stretch for a count of ten while you continue to breathe deeply, allowing your head, neck, hips, and back to relax in order to achieve the maximum full-body stretch. Slowly inhale as you gradually return to an upright position, first extending your arms straight up and then relaxing them by your sides. Perform twice.

Benefits: This exercise is especially good for runners because it stretches all the posterior muscles of the body. It also tones the abdominal viscera, keeps legs fit, and helps keep abdomen and lower back stress-free.

9. Bellows

Technique: Lie flat on your back with your arms to your sides. Relax your entire body and breathe deeply. Inhale and slowly bend your right knee, drawing it in and up toward your chest. Reach out and clasp both of your hands around the knee and hold it as close to your chest as is comfortable. Breathe deeply and hold this position for a count of ten. Then slowly exhale and

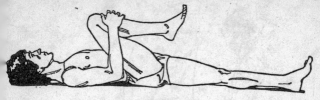

Bellows

unclasp your hands while allowing your legs to gradually straighten and lower to the floor. Relax and repeat this exercise with your left leg.

Variation 1: As your knee is clasped and drawn in to your chest, slowly raise your head off of the floor until your forehead touches your knee. Continue to breathe deeply and hold for a count of ten. Then lower your head and release your knee as in the standard stretch.

Variation 2: When your knee is to your chest, move it slowly in small circles to help loosen the muscles that connect your leg to your hip. Proceed as in the standard stretch.

Benefits: The bellows relieves stress that often accumulates in muscles surrounding the groin and pelvis during long-distance workouts. It also relieves gastrointestinal disorders such as constipation, excess gas, and indigestion. It will tone your abdominal viscera, and stretch and vitalize the muscles of the lower back, buttocks, and legs.

10. Cobra*

Technique: Lie face downward with your forehead touching the floor. Breathe normally and relax all the muscles of your body. Place your palms firmly on the floor directly below the corresponding shoulders, elbows raised slightly and close to the trunk of your body. Inhale deeply and slowly raise your head and upper half of your body. Do not move abruptly or stiffly as in a pushup. Instead, allow your head and spine to arch gracefully backward so that you can feel the stretching and bending of the vertebrae, one by one, and the pres-

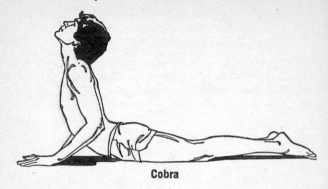

Cobra

sure traveling downward from the cervical, dorsal, and lumbar regions, and lastly to the sacral region. The lower half of your body, from navel to toes, should be still and remain resting on the floor. Breathe normally and stay in this position for a count of ten and then slowly come down, lowering the trunk first, then the head. While it is difficult to monitor breathing during this exercise, it is best to inhale while raising your body and then lower yourself on an exhalation. Perform twice.

Benefits: The cobra elasticizes all the muscles of the spine, neck, and torso and provides a healthy balance to forward bending stretches so necessary for runners. It also exercises the deep and superficial muscles of the back, allowing the spine to become supple, stretches the chest and abdomen, and aids in deepening breath and stimulating circulation. Finally, it is helpful in relieving backache and abdominal stress caused by overwork, tension, flatulence, or other common difficulties.

11. Head-to-Knee Pose*

Technique: Begin this stretch in a comfortable sitting position with your legs together and straight in front of you. Inhale and slowly stretch your arms over head. Slowly exhale, bending your entire upper body forward from the hips as you reach your hands to your toes and your chin to your knees. Breathe deeply and hold this position for a count of ten. Inhale and slowly

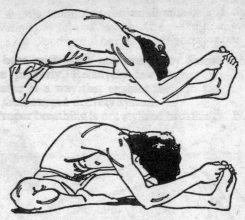

Head-to-knee pose

return to an upright sitting position with your arms once again extended straight upward. Then exhale and let your arms return to your sides. Perform twice.

Variation: As you sit comfortably upright, reach out and take hold of your right foot. Carefully bend, do *not* twist, your right knee and draw your right foot in toward your groin. Rest your right heel as close to your anus as possible. Let your right knee relax, resting as closely to the floor as is comfortable. Inhale as you slowly stretch your arms upward, exhale and slowly bend your entire upper body forward, so that your hands reach out toward your left foot, while your chin moves toward your left knee. Breathe deeply and hold this position for a count of ten. Then inhale and slowly return to an upright sitting position with your arms once again extended straight upward. Exhale and let your arms return to your sides. Carefully grasp your right foot in your hands and gently straighten your leg. Relax and repeat this exercise to the opposite side.

Benefits: This is another exercise that is especially good for runners. Like the standing forward bend, it lengthens muscles in back of the body, particularly the hamstrings of the legs and the lumbar-sacrals of the lower back. It also stimulates the abdominal viscera (liver, kidneys, and pancreas), and is helpful in trimming the waist and relaxing the neck and lower back.

12. Bow

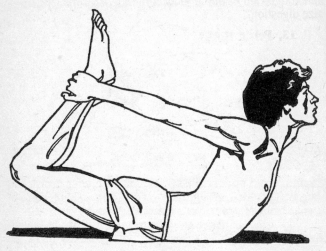

Bow

Technique: Lie face down on the floor and relax all of the muscles of your body. Bend your knees so that your feet come off of the floor and up over your thighs. Take hold of your right ankle with your right hand and your left ankle with your left hand. Inhale deeply and raise your head, trunk, and thighs off of the floor by pulling firmly on your legs with your hands. If this is done correctly the only part of your body that will remain resting on the floor will be the region between your abdomen and hips. Breathe normally and hold this position for a count of ten. (If this is difficult, you may begin by holding for a count of five.) Slowly exhale and without jerking lower your chest, head, and thighs to the floor. Then gracefully release your feet and straighten your legs to a resting position.

Benefits: The bow complements the forward bending stretches. It tones and strengthens deep and superficial muscles of back, alleviating tension and fatigue, expands the chest, deepens breathing, improves circulation, and lengthens anterior muscles of the body. It can also aid gastrointestinal functioning; alleviate dyspepsia and congestion of blood in abdominal viscera, and energize digestion.

13. Pelvic Rock*

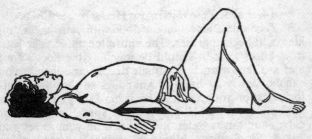

Pelvic rock—press the end of your tailbone firmly to the floor

Technique: Lie on your back and allow your entire body to relax. Breathe normally and slowly bend your knees and draw your feet along the floor until the soles are flat on the floor close to your buttocks. Press the end of your tailbone (coccyx) firmly to the floor; this will create a curvature or "hollow" in the small of your back. Then rock your pelvis back so that you are pressing the small of your back to the floor, thereby flat-

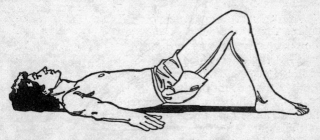

Pelvic rock—press the small of your back to the floor

tening out the hollow as your tailbone moves upward toward your knees. Breathe normally and repeat this exercise in a slow and playful rocking motion ten times.

Benefits: The pelvic rock is a good exercise to do after a workout because it relaxes the muscles in the lower back and pelvis. It also tones muscle groups in the lower back, develops intrinsic muscles of the back, pelvis, and legs, encouraging neuromuscular control, grace, and efficient body use.

14. Pelvic Pose (Sitting on Heels)

Technique: Kneel on the floor with your knees, ankles, and heels together. The entire length of your legs, from knees to toes, should be touching the floor. Your toes are gently touching. Inhale deeply, and then as you exhale, slowly sit back on your legs so that your buttocks rest on your heels. If this is hard for you to do, begin by placing a small pillow in the space between your calves and thighs to lessen the stress on your knees and ankles. Sit comfortably upright so that you are looking forward with your trunk, head and neck in a straight

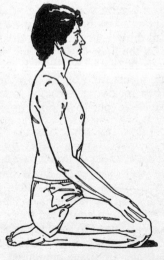

Pelvic pose

line. Place your hands palms down over your knees and allow your shoulders and back to relax fully. Breathe normally, still your thoughts, and hold this position for a count of 20. Then slowly stand up, shake out your legs, and repeat.

Benefits: This exercise works to loosen up joints, tendons, and ligaments in legs which grow stiff and fragile from regular workouts and distance running. It strengthens legs and thighs; tones ankle and knee joints.

15. Spinal Roll*

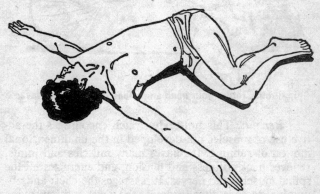

Spinal roll—bend your knees and draw them upward to your chest

Technique: Lie comfortably on your back and relax all of the muscles of your body. Breathe normally and extend your arms outward on the floor so that they rest perpendicular to your spine. Slowly bend your knees and draw them upward to approximately 5 inches from your chest. Your heels should be close to your buttocks which are also slightly raised. Then breathe deeply and rotate your lower body to the right side as you gently turn your head to the left side. Allow your buttocks and head to turn as far as is comfortable. Then slowly return your head and knees to center and reverse directions. Continue breathing normally and repeat this motion five times on each side.

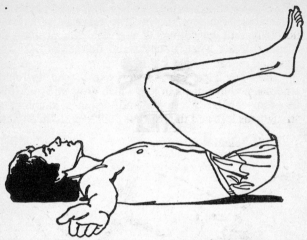

Spinal roll—return your head and knees to center and reverse

Benefits: This full-body stretch encourages the active use of muscles not developed in the unidimensional motion of running. It relaxes many muscles and joints, relieves neck stiffness and tension, and energizes all the spinal muscles and nerves. It massages the chest and abdominal regions, thus trimming the waist and improving circulation, breathing, and digestion.

16. Shoulder Stand

Technique: Lie flat on your back, palms downward alongside your body. Inhale and slowly raise your legs until they are perpendicular to the floor. Continue raising your legs, hips, and trunk to a vertical position, while simultaneously raising your forearms and positioning your hands on your lower back for support. Press your chin against your chest and allow your entire body from neck to toes to be as relaxed and straight as possible. While holding this position, the back of your head, neck, shoulders, upper arms, and elbows should rest firmly on the floor. Breathe normally and hold this position for a count of 15. To come down, exhale and let go of your back and allow it to gracefully return to

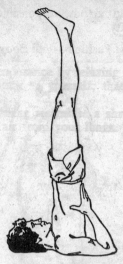

Shoulder stand

the floor. Then gently lower your legs to the floor and return to a relaxed lying position.

Variation: If this position is difficult for you to assume comfortably, many of the same benefits can be received by performing a modified version of the shoulder stand. For example, with your legs elevated you can position yourself on your back with your buttocks close to a wall and then slide your legs upward from the side until they are perpendicular to the floor, feet resting on the wall. Hold this position for several minutes. Be sure to relax and breathe deeply while holding this posture.

Benefits: The shoulder stand reverses the effect of gravity on the cardiovascular system: it returns the blood more easily to the heart for purification, and pumps blood to the neck and head to energize the brain and scalp. As a result, lymphatic toxins stored in the legs are gently released, cleansing the body's waste disposal system. Shoulder stands free up internal organs, improving gastrointestinal functioning. They focus an enormous amount of energy and blood on the thyroid and parathyroid glands, responsible for maintaining metabolic vitality.

17. Corpse Position—Full Body Relaxation*

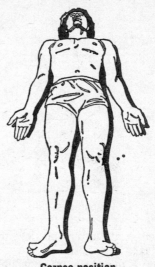

Corpse position

Technique: Lie on your back with your feet relaxed and spread several inches apart and your arms alongside your body palms upward. Close your eyes and allow your entire body to relax and rest. Focus your mind on your deep and regular breathing, while releasing any stress or tension. Practice full yogic breathing and hold this pose for several minutes. This exercise can be performed after running, or at any other time during the day, in order to release stress and allow the body to refresh itself.

Benefits: This is perhaps the most important of all exercises: an excellent vehicle for stress reduction as well as physical and mental relaxation. It allows the body-mind to clear itself of tension, fatigue, and stress and thereby revitalize itself.

VI

The Physiology of Running Right

Running produces a rich variety of physical sensations, some of them pleasant, some of them not so pleasant, but most of them fairly universal. Much of the time, the origins of these sensations are obvious. You don't have to be a biologist or exercise physiologist, for instance, to understand why you perspire when you run, why you get thirsty, and why you can get winded if you try to run beyond your capacity.

But other physical properties of running don't lend themselves to easy explanations. Why is it, for example, that you can start out on a run one morning feeling stiff and sluggish and convinced you're never going to survive the first 400 yards, only to find that moments later you're running better and more effortlessly than you've ever run? And how many times has the exact opposite happened: you start out feeling fresh and strong and loose only to turn in one of the worst running performances of your life?

What about all those other experiences that runners talk about? Second wind. Is there such a thing, and what explains it? And how about the "wall"?

What is really happening in your body when you run into the "wall"? And how inevitable is it?

If you're like most runners, you've probably never given much thought to any of these questions. You probably figure that your body is going to react in certain ways regardless of how much you understand what's going on, so why concern yourself; why not leave well enough alone?

Well, I don't share this outlook. Not at all. There's a very good and very basic reason for developing an understanding of just what goes on inside your body at different stages of a run. Every physical sensation you experience when you run represents a message from your body that tells you what is happening, and once you understand this language, you can then manage your running all the more effectively. You'll be able to tell when you can—and can't—reach down for energy. You'll be able to recognize when something is wrong and you're better off stopping. By developing this awareness of what is happening inside your body when you run, you'll be arming yourself with a mental weapon that will help you run with more confidence. It's the old story of knowledge being power, and it's just as true of running as it is of other disciplines.

So what I'm going to try to do in this chapter is present a picture of the physiological processes that underlie the physical sensations we all experience when we run. I should emphasize here that exercise physiology, in and of itself, is a complex field and there is not only much that is not known but much that is debated about what *is* known. I myself am no expert in exercise physiology. I've tried to put together a picture that represents the sum of what is generally accepted by certain members of the scientific community and what has been borne out by personal experience. As recently as five years ago, I couldn't have begun to write on this subject with any degree of certainty, and it's reasonable to suggest that in another five years much of what I say here will be superseded by additional knowledge.

The Basics of Running

We run with more than just our legs. We run with our lungs, our hearts, our livers, our nervous systems. Indeed, there isn't a major organ or major system in the body that doesn't affect the running experience one way or the other.

To describe in detail the physiological role played by every part of the body would take a book unto itself, so we're going to focus our attention chiefly on the systems and the body components that play the most direct role in determining how well we run, how long we run, and how comfortably we run. In particular, we'll be looking into the activity that takes place inside individual muscle cells. By familiarizing yourself with what is going on at the cellular level when you run, you can gain insight into the overall physiological picture of running, and you can use this information to help you train better and run better.

Energy Production in the Cell

Running takes energy. Energy is burned at the cellular level. Carbohydrates are the body's prime energy source. When carbohydrates get depleted (as in a long run), then the body burns fatty acids for energy. When there are no more fatty acids left to burn, the body utilizes protein. This is why runners eat spaghetti the night before long runs instead of steak.

The burning of energy takes place in the mitochondria, the "powerhouse" of the cell. It is here in the mitochondria that energy sources are broken down (through metabolism) into ATP (adenosine triphosphate) molecules. The name of the running game is producing ATP's efficiently and in abundance. Production of ATP's creates the energy which causes the contractions in the muscles which propel the runner.

Though energy is produced in the cells, the cells are dependent upon the bloodstream to provide the necessary ingredients (especially oxygen), for maximum energy production. The bloodstream also serves the vital function of removing the waste products which are a result of ATP production.

So, when we're talking about the physiology of running, we're concerned primarily with two functions: one, the work performed by individual cells; and, two, the ability of the rest of the body to deliver the raw material—nutrients, oxygen, etc.—that enables the cells to perform work. Certainly there are other physiological aspects of running, but these are the two most crucial, and these are the two we'll be looking into in detail in this chapter.

Producing ATP

Muscle cells have several different ways of producing and utilizing ATP. In the first place, a small supply of ATP is always kept in storage during periods of rest. This reservoir of energy, however, is in a slightly different form—a chemical bond known as creatine phosphate (CP). This reservoir of energy is limited: it can provide the energy needed for hard muscle work for no more than a few seconds. So while it is useful—especially for sprinters—its value to a long-distance runner is minor.

Once CP reserves are gone, the cell must synthesize new ATP. It does this by extracting nutrients—chiefly glucose—from the bloodstream and converting them into ATP. It has two methods of doing this. One method, known as glycolysis, accomplishes the production of ATP without oxygen—that is, anaerobically. The other method, known as the Krebs cycle, accomplishes the conversion using oxygen—that is, aerobically. Whether a cell produces ATP anaerobically or aerobically depends entirely on the amount of oxygen available to the cell. When the oxygen supply is sufficient to meet the energy needs of the cell, the cell will produce ATP aerobically. When there isn't enough oxygen available, the cell will go into an anaerobic production cycle.

Aerobics and Anaerobics: The Difference

Most runners associate aerobic and anaerobic running with how comfortable you feel when you run. If you're able to breathe comfortably when you run you are running aerobically, and when you're out of breath you are in an anaerobic state.

But the true picture is considerably more complex for the difference between aerobic and anaerobic running isn't so much how you feel, but rather how your body is processing energy. As long as there is a sufficient supply of oxygen to meet your body's energy needs you are in an aerobic state. But when there isn't enough oxygen your body seeks alternate sources, which we'll get to in a moment.

The main thing to remember though, is that aerobic and anaerobic are terms that relate to what is happening at a cellular level, and not necessarily what you are consciously experiencing. Inhaling more oxygen (say from an oxygen tank) when your lungs are laboring during anaerobic phases won't instantly put you back into an aerobic state for the blood needs time to carry the oxygen to the working cells. All of which reinforces the importance of an efficient cardiovascular system for efficient running.

Given the fact that muscle cells can produce ATP's with or without oxygen, it is reasonable to wonder whether or not it makes any difference; it does. The differences concern efficiency—and what is important to the runner, the elimination of waste materials such as carbon dioxide and lactic acid which can cause so much pain and discomfort during a run.

Broadly speaking, the picture is as follows:

A certain amount of anaerobic metabolism (glycolysis) occurs all the time. During normal aerobic metabolism about 38 units of ATP are produced. When there is insufficient oxygen, glycolysis plays a major role and only two units of ATP are produced. As you can see, glycolysis is a very inefficient means of producing energy.

There is a logic behind these differences. There are, after all, certain physical activities—a sprint, weight lifting—in which you need to generate all-out exertion for a short period of time. Glycolysis provides ample energy for these short bursts. But in other activities, such as long distance running, the need for concentrated short bursts of energy isn't as great. Distance runners, therefore, need to build up their aerobic capacities.

Hence the difference: anaerobic processing for short bursts of all-out activity; aerobic processing for sustained activity. There are definite limits to the body's anaerobic capacity. Even a well-conditioned athlete can sustain an all-out anaerobic effort for only a few seconds. At this point, a combination of factors—the heating up of the cell, the accumulation of waste products around the cell—compromise the cell's ability to extract nutrients from the bloodstream. Until a more normal environment returns, the cell cannot resume functioning properly.

It is true that through training you can improve the anaerobic capacity of your muscles, but only to a degree. Regardless of how much you train and how well conditioned you are, there comes a time during glycolysis when the raw fuel supply is no longer available. At this stage, the cell can do only one of two things: it can stop working, or if there is enough oxygen available it can begin to synthesize ATP through the aerobically powered Krebs cycle.

Aerobic Processing and Oxygen

Like glycolysis, aerobic metabolism in the cell originates with the extraction of glucose from the bloodstream. But with oxygen present the chemical scenario changes. As we've just seen, glycolysis uses only about 5 percent of the energy potential of the glucose molecule. The chief by-product of glycolysis is pyruvic acid. What we generally think of as aerobic processing begins with the conversion of pyruvic acid molecules into acetyl-CoA. The key step in the Krebs cycle involves the freeing of hydrogen atoms from the acetyl-CoA molecule. These hydrogen atoms ultimately combine with oxygen to form water, and it is during this symbiotic meeting that the ATP molecules are formed.

But enough chemistry. The thing you want to bear in mind about aerobic energy processing is that it is a much more efficient means of producing ATP than glycolysis—it makes far more productive use of raw energy. What's more, the aerobic reactions that take place during the Krebs cycle also make use of the chemical energy contained in other nutrients, namely other sugars, fats, and proteins. There are a couple of drawbacks to this rosy picture. For one thing, aerobic processing requires the presence of oxygen. Second, as we've already seen, it's a more time-consuming process than glycolysis.

Getting Oxygen Into the Energy Act

If you've read any of the many running books on the market today, you've undoubtedly run into the phrase "aerobic capacity." What the phrase means, in brief, is the ability of your body's oxygen intake and transport system to supply enough energy so that the cells can operate aerobically.

It's impossible to be in an aerobic state throughout the full course of a run. But there are other reasons it's next to impossible to run entirely in an aerobic state. Let's assume you're midway through a 5-mile run. If you're running at, say, an eight-minute-per-mile rate, you've probably been in an aerobic state since about halfway into your first mile. You're running comfortably. Your cells are getting the oxygen they need. ATP production is moving along in fine shape. But now you come to a steep hill. If you're going to maintain your pace, you have to force the muscles to work harder. By forcing the muscles to work harder, you increase the oxygen demand, and if your oxygen delivery system isn't equal to the task, you'll run into a temporary shortage of oxygen. You have two options: you can slow down your pace so that you regain the balance between oxygen supply and oxygen need, or you can continue to work the muscles vigorously, producing an oxygen deficit which, in turns, triggers a return to anaerobic processing. You'll have to work harder in the anaerobic state, and you may experience discomfort, but for a time at least you can run even though there isn't enough oxygen in the cells to supply present energy needs.

During a run you may slip in and out of anaerobic and aerobic states, depending on the degree to which your oxygen delivery system can keep the cells supplied with enough oxygen to meet basic energy needs. The key to successful distance running is to minimize the amount of time you're forced to run anaerobically (a good marathoner, for instance, will run the 26.2 miles 95 percent aerobically and only 5 percent anaerobically). Your capacity to run well can be improved through proper training.

Transporting the Energy

Before your muscle cells can convert raw nutrients into ATP, it has to receive these nutrients. Here is where the bloodstream enters the picture.

The bloodstream carries not only food nutrients but oxygen to cells. Oxygen is transported from the lungs to the muscle tissues via the tiny red blood cells called hemoglobin. Hemoglobin is a little like a railroad tank car. Having a great affinity for oxygen, the hemoglobin loads up as much as it can store and then heads immediately for the areas of the body that require the most oxygen. The body is remarkably adept at sending oxygen where it is most needed. Right after a meal, for instance, the bulk of the available oxygen gets sent to the digestive tract to help the cells do their work. During periods of heavy exercise, oxygen heads directly to the muscles being used.

Once the oxygen-heavy hemoglobin reaches the needy cell, it gives up its load to the so-called oxygen storehouse of the muscle cell—myoglobin. Like hemoglobin, myoglobin is an iron-rich protein with a great affinity for oxygen. The difference, though, is that myoglobin is permanently fixed to the cell. The myoglobin relieves the hemoglobin of its energy load, and the hemoglobin is reloaded with carbon dioxide waste.

Not too long ago, trainers and exercise physiologists pretty much ignored what happened to hemoglobin once it delivered its load of oxygen to needy cells. But recent research shows that the body's ability to get rid of chemical waste products—chiefly, carbon dioxide—may be as crucial to running performance as its ability to deliver oxygen.

What happens to this waste is very important to the runner. The hemoglobin transports carbon dioxide out through the veins, into the heart, out into the lungs, and it is expelled by the body via exhalation of breath. There are some researchers who feel that this is the key to long distance endurance. They refer to it as the ability to run with *carbon dioxide tension*. While some say that the most important aspect in endurance is getting enough oxygen to the cells in order to prevent anaerobia from setting in, a growing minority feels that there is always enough oxygen present. They feel that it is the inability of the body to get rid of the waste (mainly carbon dioxide) quickly that causes all the problems. The waste causes excessive acidity which interferes with efficient ATP production. Though it sounds like two sides of the same coin, this difference is vital to serious runners.

This discovery has triggered a number of new training concepts that we'll talk about a little later.

The Power Behind the System

Every system needs a power source, including your body's energy transport system. Whether you are operating in an aerobic or anaerobic state, the power source behind the transport system is the same: it is the heart.

The basic function of the heart is to pump blood throughout the body. The heart is nothing more than a muscle. Like leg muscles, the heart needs energy to function efficiently. The more efficiently the heart works, the more blood it can pump in a single beat.

When we talk about heart rate, we're talking about the number of times the heart beats per minute. It is one of the basic principles of exercise physiology that the more efficient your cardiovascular system is, the lower your heart rate will be. Kenneth Cooper has pointed out that the heart of a person in good cardiovascular condition is likely to beat as many as 500 *fewer* times per day than the heart of a person in average condition.

Powerful as it is, the heart can only pump so many times per minute. In extreme circumstances the heart has been known to register 220 beats per minute. This is neither normal, nor beneficial. Each of us has a maximum heart rate—the maximum number of beats per minute the heart is capable of logging during strenuous exercise.

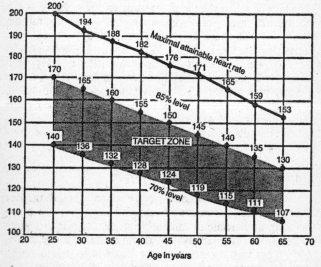

MAXIMUM ATTAINABLE HEART RATE AND TARGET ZONE

Age affects maximum heart rate. As a general guide, in order to calculate a normal heart rate, subtract your age from 220. If you are thirty years old, your maximum heart rate will be 190. If you are 42 years old it will be 178 and so forth.

Now that you know your maximum heart rate, it is vital that you know your exercise heart range. Learning to operate within this exercise heart range is your key to improved conditioning.

Your exercise heart range is the number of beats per minute which indicate the optimum level of stress you can subject your body to in order to cause a positive physical adaptation.

This rate varies according to age, but for most people it's anywhere between 120 and 180 beats per minute. Let's say you are 30 years old. If you look at the chart you'll see that your exercise heart range is between 136 and 165. So if your heart is beating less than 136 per minute you are not stressing the adaptive mechanisms in your body enough to make any difference in your fitness level. But at the same time, an over 165 heart beat rate is not going to help you too much either, since your heart is probably unable to either fill up completely or empty completely.

All of which again underscores the importance of heart function to running. For not only is it important for hemoglobin to get oxygen to the working muscles quickly and efficiently, but equally (if not more) important to get enough oxygen to the most important muscle of them all—the heart. How the heart utilizes oxygen and the conserved energy in ATP bonds is not fully understood. A working leg muscle may contract 75 times in a minute, and as we have seen, it's plenty difficult getting enough oxygen and an adequate food supply to enable this amount of work to take place. Yet the muscles of the heart may be contracting at 175 beats per minute, over twice as fast as a leg muscle. How the heart functions under these conditions for long periods of time is nothing shot of miraculous.

What Happens Physiologically When You Run

Now that you have a general idea of the general physiological principles that underlie running, let's try to connect some of these principles to the actual running experience.

We'll start at the beginning: when you start your run. Earlier we talked about the reservoir of energy, CP. This source of ATP is limited but you can increase the amount of time it lasts you by controlling your pace. The biggest mistake that recreational runners make in fun runs or real races is to start too fast. Quick starts demand a lot of energy quickly. CP is there to support the initial burst, but if it gets used up too quickly, your cells are forced to switch to anaerobic processing. This wouldn't be too bad if it weren't for one aspect of anaerobic metabolizing we haven't yet talked about that deserves a close look: lactic acid.

Lactic acid is a chemical by-product of glycolysis. Though some lactate is being produced at all times, when the concentration of lactic acid surpasses the body's ability to break it down, it causes the area around the cells to become very acidic. Soon the enzymes are unable to perform their metabolic functions and the whole system breaks down.

If you exercise vigorously, you are not a stranger to the discomfort caused by lactic acid. It can cause stiffness, that aching sense of fatigue, and sometimes severe pain.

On the other hand, lactic acid is actually a sheep in wolf's clothing. For in long runs it is more of an ally than an enemy. The body is continually rushing that lactic acid through the bloodstream, back to the liver where it is oxidized, and returns to the system in glycogen form as a secondary energy source!

Though nobody knows for certain, this phenomenon might be the cause of what is commonly called "second-wind." It is possible that the sudden, unexplained burst of energy you sometimes feel during a long race is quite simply your body being revitalized by a fresh energy source—the glycogen which is in reality recycled lactic acid.

Maximal Oxygen Intake

Sustained activity exhausts the capacity of the muscle cell to produce ATP through glycolysis in a relatively short time. If the activity is to continue, the cell needs oxygen, which brings us to two physiological functions central to running: (1) oxygen consumption, the amount of oxygen that is used up during the metabolism process in the cells, and (2) the oxygen transport system, consisting of the heart, veins, arteries, capillaries, and blood plasma—in short, all the elements involved in getting the oxygen where it is needed and then ridding the body of the waste that is the result of the energy-producing activity inside the cells.

Maximum oxygen consumption refers to the point at which your oxygen intake and delivery system can no longer keep pace with the oxygen demands of your working cells. This level differs considerably from person to person. The idea of measuring this capacity was popularized by Dr. Kenneth Cooper in his book *Aerobics*. The basic notion is that the distance you can run in 12 minutes, or the time it takes you to run 1.5 miles, are fairly accurate measures of your oxygen consumption capacity. Obviously, the higher your rate of oxygen consumption, the more easily you can maintain aerobic energy production.

What are the bodily factors that affect your maximum consumption rate? According to E. C. Frederick, they are the following:

1. The rate at which your lungs can take in and exhale air, and the volume of air that can be handled in a given time.

2. The capacity of the blood—specifically, of hemoglobin—to carry oxygen.

3. The ability of the heart and peripheral circulatory system to transport oxygenated blood to the tissues.

4. The capacity of the blood to give up oxygen and of the cell tissues to bind oxygen once it gets delivered to the cells.

5. The capacity of the individual cells to utilize oxygen in the production of ATP molecules.

Most exercise physiologists consider the maximum oxygen consumption rate the single most reliable indicator of running performance. Most long-distance training is based on the idea of increasing this capacity. But as we become more sophisticated in our training methods, we're beginning to see that there is more to an outstanding running performance than your maximum oxygen consumption rate. Dr. David Costill, of Ball State College, for example, has done some impressive research that shows that more than maximum oxygen consumption rate, it's the ability to maintain a high percentage of maximum oxygen consumption rate over a long period of time that separates the runners from the plodders in high-level competition.

No matter how high your oxygen consumption level is, the trick is to be able to utilize 100 percent of it during a long run. Most runners don't; they use less and less of potential capacity as the race goes on. A recreational runner, for example, may be using 80 percent of his capacity during the first few miles of a ten-mile run; by the seventh or eighth mile he may be using less than 50 percent of his capacity.

If you take two runners, measure their maximum oxygen consumption capacity, and pit them against each other, assuming that variables such as stride length, fiber twitch (an indication of innate speed potential), anaerobic capacity, cardiovascular system, and mental states are somewhat alike, in shorter races of 3 miles or less, with both runners using close to 100 percent of their MOC capacity, they would be about equally likely to win. But in races of 5, 10, 15 miles and more, the odds favor the runner with the ability to maintain a higher percentage of his MOC capacity for a prolonged period of time.

This distinction can have an important bearing on the kind of training you do. Nobody disputes that the best way to improve your maximum oxygen capacity is through long and sustained periods of aerobic running—"LSD training." But there is no conclusive evidence that LSD training is better than other methods, such as interval training, for building up your ability to sustain MOC for over a long period of time.

Beefing Up Hemoglobin

Just as myoglobin levels can be increased through training, the amount of hemoglobin in the bloodstream can be increased. It has been proved that training in high altitude, for instance, though it does not increase oxygen consumption, as originally thought, does increase the amount of hemoglobin in the blood. Obviously, the more hemoglobin is available to carry oxygen from the lungs to the muscle tissue, the more oxygen is going to arrive where it is needed most.

The importance of hemoglobin levels may be of special interest to cigarette smokers. Besides the damage that inhaled smoke does to the cilia of the bronchi and the lungs, smoking also affects hemoglobin transport of oxygen. Hemoglobin, it seems, has an even higher affinity for the carbon monoxide gas contained in cigarette smoke than it does for oxygen. Some researchers think that the carbon monoxide gas literally shatters the hemoglobin, but other evidence suggests that the hemoglobin accepts the carbon monoxide gas instead of the beneficial oxygen. Either way, carbon monoxide leaves less hemoglobin free for the all-important task of getting oxygen where it is needed the most. A pack of cigarettes a day can reduce the capacity of your oxygen transport system by 7 to 10 percent.

Up Against the "Wall"

If we only needed a steady supply of oxygen to keep a cell functioning, we could, in theory, train ourselves to run forever. But oxygen, remember, is only a catalyzing agent in the energy production process. It is only an energy source when it interacts with nutrients that come from either the food we eat or the body's energy reserves.

One of the limits we face when we run is the supply of nutrients in the body. Different nutrients are necessary for different body functions. When it comes to energy processing, carbohydrates are the most important energy source. The reason is that carbohydrates, which get broken down into simple sugars as soon as they enter the digestive tract, are the simplest molecules in the food chain and the easiest for the cells to break down.

There is enough material in other books to explain how nutrients get broken down and eventually make their way to the cell, but there is one aspect of the process that warrants special attention: namely, what happens when the body's supply of carbohydrates gets used up but you still need energy.

In this case the body switches to a new energy source—the fatty acids stored in the liver in the form of glycogen. There is both good news and bad in this area of energy metabolism. The good news is that these fatty acids, once converted, are a rich form of energy—a third more rich in ATP potential than glucose and 25 times as rich in ATP potential as glucose during glycolysis. The bad news is that the waste products that result from the metabolizing of these fatty acids can cause you a great deal of discomfort. The waste products are called ketone bodies and they produce a condition of acidity around the cell known as ketosis. Ketone body buildup is to lactic acid buildup what 180-proof grain alcohol is to a glass of sherry. The heavy acidity can be so great, in fact, that joints freeze up and cease to function. This is the pain that marathon runners experience routinely. Yes, there is a "wall." So while there are energy sources beyond carbohydrates, and while they are a rich source of energy, relying on them is a little like dealing with loan sharks. They'll provide you what you need—ready energy—but they'll exact a painfully high rate of interest.

Cooling Down

The more energy your body consumes, the hotter it gets. The reason at the cellular level is that ATP production increases the temperature of the muscle cell.

As the cells heat up, acid develops around them, making it more difficult for them to extract the nutrients needed for ATP production. So it's essential that the body have a way of regulating the temperature environment around cells, of keeping this environment in balance so that energy production can go on.

The body can do this, but it's not easy—particularly when you put yourself through the rigors of a long-distance run. The body's method of cooling down cells is to secrete body fluids. The body takes the heat generated from the body cells and carries it to the capillaries close to the skin surface, where excess heat seeps into the atmosphere in the form of perspiration.

But in order to perform this cooling-off function, the body needs plenty of fluids. This is why, in a long race, you have to be particularly concerned about the possibility of dehydration, especially when you're running in humid conditions. With high humidity in the air, the perspiration that reaches the skin surface can't evaporate into the atmosphere easily, so instead of being released at the skin level, it remains in a liquid state and fails to help cool the blood.

Nearly all the fluid lost in a long race is water that comes from the intracellular spaces. As long as there is enough water in these spaces to cool the body, you don't have to concern yourself too much with body temperature, but when the supply of water dries up the result is dehydration.

More important perhaps than fluid loss is the loss of electrolytes that goes with it: ions of sodium, potassium, calcium, and magnesium, without which nerve functions will not operate properly. We haven't talked much about the specifics of neural control of muscles, but the cells involved—neurons—require a specific balance of ions in order to give and receive the coded impulses which direct the internal actions of the body. When this delicate balance is upset, the body compensates by ceasing to function in certain areas. Cramps set in, and your general coordination is hampered.

This is why a "runners' punch" is so important during, say, a marathon. Whether it is ERG, actionade, Gatorade, or a homemade concoction, so long as it is rich in potassium, magnesium, and sodium, this potent brew will surely aid any marathoner during the long ordeal. Researchers disagree on whether magnesium or potassium is the most important ion to be ingested, but everyone agrees that in any race of more than an hour, it is a good idea to take in some sort of fluid that is rich in electrolytes.

Another important point to bear in mind when you run on a hot day is to drink fluids even if you're not thirsty. Researchers have lately found that the thirst mechanism is not adequate to maintain a reasonable electrolyte balance. So if you are running in a race of an hour or more, don't wait until you get thirsty to begin drinking an electrolyte solution. And don't increase your intake with the idea of loading up. Large amounts at one time are likely to upset your stomach.

The best thing to do is to drink small amounts all along the route. If you are a conditioned runner, you should be able to drink 12 ounces of an electrolyte solution before starting a race. Then, if it is permitted, should begin your gradual intake of electrolytes at the 4- or 5-mile mark. *If you wait until you are really thirsty for refreshments, it will be too late to make up the electrolyte loss already suffered.*

Physiology and Training Practices

I have gone into such detail in describing some of the physiological aspects of running not only to familiarize you with these processes but to put you in a better position to follow a more intelligent training pattern. Granted, much of what we've discussed concerns microscopic activity whose control is far beyond the limits of our current knowledge. We know of no way yet that you can increase the number of ATP molecules that can be produced during glycolysis. We know of no way that you can minimize the excretion of waste products when your body switches energy sources from carbohydrates to fatty acids. We know of no way you can control the delicate balance of electrolytes. With proper mental training, people can already raise and lower their heart rates at will. Perhaps we are not far from gaining mental control over cellular activity. So, by tomorrow's standards our training methods may be crude. Who knows but that in 20 years or so, runners will be gearing their workouts to units of ATP produced by glycolysis per minute?

All the same, our methods of training are much more sophisticated than they have ever been. We know, for example, that while you can't postpone the onset of anaerobia indefinitely, you can train your body to forestall it. And we know that you can bring about an overall increase in the body's ability to take in and deliver oxygen. This brings us back to the heart.

Some superbly conditioned marathon runners have recorded sustained heartbeats of 95 percent of their maximum heart rate, so that a runner with a maximum pulse of 190 beats per minute can sustain a rate of 181 beats for the duration of a marathon (26.2 miles), which is 2½ to 3 hours. Since oxygen consumption correlates closely with cardiac output and heart rate, it is safe to say that this runner is getting about all from his body that it has to give, at least physically.

Naturally, such a highly efficient running body requires a massive arterial and capillary system if it is to keep up with the oxygen demand of such stressful situations, a system that can be enlarged through proper training. The number of arteries can be increased, along with the size of the capillaries, which permits more oxygen rich blood to pass through them. As you might guess, the muscles you use the most are the chief beneficiaries of the increased capacity of your arterial and capillary systems. The calf muscle, for example, is capable of doubling its capillary density as the result of a rigorous running program.

No one knows for sure, but the suspicion is that these arterial and capillary systems increase their size and number not individually but in groups or large networks. This may be why training seems to progress in plateau fashion. We have all experienced this. We run for a while, notice improvement, then seem to stagnate. All of a sudden, we take a quantum leap forward. One theory holds that these leaps forward result from the opening up of new arterial and capillary networks. Once these networks begin functioning to their full capacity, the working muscles receive more oxygen for aerobic respiration, and the carbon dioxide waste gets carried away faster.

But the converse is apt to be true. If your training is not conducive (after an initial stage) to the rapid expansion of arterial and capillary systems, it is conceivable that day-to-day running will yield less noticeable improvement than when you first started out. And regardless of your training schedule, your rate of improvement will always decline after the initial stages.

So it is not difficult to appreciate the physiological effects that training has on the human body. The way you train effects every part of your system, right down to the cellular level. Training affects your maximum oxygen uptake and maximum breathing capacity, the volume of blood, the number of red blood cells and the amount of hemoglobin in those cells; the increase in hemoglobin in turn increases the amount of oxygen that can be transported from the lungs to the working cells. Training increases the carrying capacity of the actual channels of transportation, the arteries and capillaries. It raises the capacity of myoglobin (the cell's storehouse); it improves the efficiency of the mitochondria (the powerhouse inside the cell). Training even increases the quantity of enzymes that make up the Krebs cycle and the electron transfer system, so that these cycles operate more smoothly; and, of course, training increases the size and efficiency of the heart dramatically, so that it not only pumps more blood with each beat when you run, it lowers the number of beats required to produce the volume of blood you need. The result: your cells get more oxygen to use as fuel, producing more ATP and providing more energy for more muscle contractions before anaerobia sets in. You achieve more work with less effort. You run faster and longer with less pain.

VII

Variety

The jogger, for example, can run a mile in eight minutes every day for a year. At the end of the year, he will be in worse shape than he was at the end of the second month. For the first two months, running a mile would improve his condition. But if he continues to run the mile in exactly the same way, he will adapt to that demand, his response will diminish and he will begin to "decondition."

—LAURENCE MOREHOUSE, M.D.

If I had my way, every jogger would have this quote from *Total Fitness* pasted on his or her mirror. It dramatizes a point that coaches and seasoned runners take for granted, but a point most recreational runners don't appreciate at all. It points up the crucial role that variety plays in the training routine of a runner.

Variety serves two important functions: (1) it helps you cope with boredom; (2) it improves your running.

As I pointed out in chapter I, it has been the development of imaginative training systems using a variety of training techniques that has accounted for the remarkable improvement in times of competitive runners. The use of these techniques helps prevent the problems that Dr. Morehouse cites, of the body accommodating to a physical routine that doesn't change. The whole purpose of training is to counteract this tendency, to maintain—at a reasonable level—enough stresses on the body to produce conditioning. Stress forces the body to adapt, producing an increase in work capacity. For the runner, this means an increase in strength and endurance. There are limits, of course, but most people —certainly most recreational runners—are in no danger of exceeding them.

This is why I am convinced that the training regimen for any runner must consist of a variety of running approaches. The approaches I'm talking about can be broken down into three categories:

1. Long Continuous Distance Running (LCD): For improving maximum oxygen uptake and aerobic metabolism, and for conditioning your body to use fatty acids as an energy source once carbohydrate stores have been depleted.

2. Interval Training: To improve anaerobic metabolism, which means helping your cardiovascular system to bring nutrients to the working tissue more efficiently and to carry away waste products more quickly.

3. Resistance Training: To strengthen leg muscles, to increase the body's tolerance of lactic acid, and to stress the cardiovascular system.

Regardless of whether you do LCD, interval, or resistance running, you will only realize the true advantages of variety if you vary the *tempo* of the run, and the *gait*.

"Gait" describes a particular style of movement used in running. Tempo refers to how much effort (or how fast) you run using that particular style of motion. The gait is how you run. Tempo is how fast you run. The gaits and tempos used in my program (from slowest to fastest) are:

GAIT	TEMPO (% of Effort)	PERCENT OF MAXIMUM HEART RATE
Shuffle	15%	Below 70
Fresh Swing	15–50%	65–75
Good Swing	50–85%	75–80
Good Speed	50 (different motion)	75
Sprint	85–100%	80–100

Chances are that in your current workouts you either run at a sprint or jog. Varied gaits will add sophistication to your running repertory. These gaits have the added advantage of being geared to your exercise heart range, which means you won't have to check your pulse every two minutes. The shuffle, for example, is done at well below 70 percent of your maximum heart range (cardiac threshold), while good swing is done at the upper levels. So once you familiarize yourself with the style of motion, you can exercise in the proper heart range without even looking at a watch.

Take two days to familiarize yourself with these techniques. A smooth grass field about 100 yards long is probably the best area for this preparation.

Shuffle

The shuffle is the slowest gait, requiring no more than 15 percent of your maximum effort. It was developed by Bill Emmerton, a Tasmanian who is best known for his runs across Death Valley, and for his historic run from Houston to Cape Kennedy to commemorate the first moon launching. (He averaged 50 miles a day for 28 days.) There's nothing complicated about the shuffle: it is a slow-paced run with the feet kept close to the ground. Emmerton's advice is to concentrate your awareness below your knees, landing on your heels and pushing out from your knees. It helps, too, to keep your arms low, which cuts down on the effort needed to carry you forward.

The shuffle is good to use on a long continuous run. Be careful to keep below 15 percent effort; otherwise you'll end up with sore shins and calves. This gait

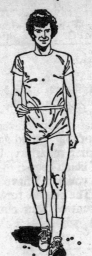

Shuffle—front view

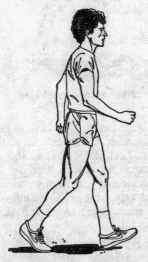

Shuffle—side view

should be used primarily for warming up, for beginning slow aerobic runs, and for slowing down when fatigued.

Fresh Swing

The fresh swing gait is done by lifting your knees slightly higher than you did for the shuffle and by step-

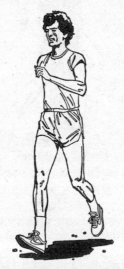

Fresh swing—front view

ping out into a large stride. You have to pay attention to where your foot lands. Chances are, your natural foot plant is near the heel, somewhat to the outside of the foot. Don't change this natural step, but allow yourself to roll off the outside of your foot toward the middle. If you do this correctly, you get a feeling of rolling from one foot to the next. Don't overemphasize! Just follow the natural foot fall.

This easy flowing gait should be run anywhere from 15 to 50% of a sprint. If you find yourself out of breath, you're going too fast.

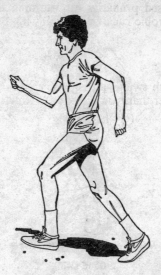

Fresh swing—side view

Good Swing

Good swing is similar to fresh swing, only it is a bit faster. You plant your foot a little farther up toward the toe, and the stride is somewhat longer. If you don't find yourself getting out of breath (becoming anaerobic), you are going too slow.

Good Speed

The object of Igloi's good speed gait is to change your running rhythm so that you use less muscles. The good speed gait conserves energy. In good speed your step is shorter, your knee lift is higher, and your foot plant is near the heels. What's more (this is the key), the arm swing is from side to side, as though you were using two hands to dust back and forth across a table.

If you use this gait you may resemble a child running. This isn't bad. Cerutty often said, "Watch a child run and do likewise."

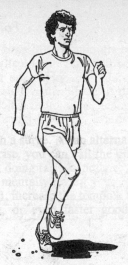

Good swing

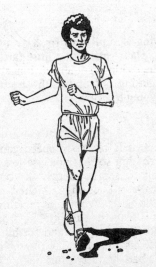

Good speed

Acceleration and Junction Point

If you are running a 200-yard interval, and you want to run the first half aerobically and the last 100 yards anaerobically, you begin the run in fresh swing and then switch to good swing. This build up is called an acceleration, and the point at which you change from one gait to another is called the junction point.

Igloi liked to use the restorative motion of good speed for a quick change in momentum at midpoint in a run or when driving toward the finish line. Sometimes he'd call for the change at a junction point. Sometimes he'd order a whole set run in good speed, sandwiched between fresh swing tempos. The purpose of the change in momentum was to endow the run with freshness.

Skip Shake-up

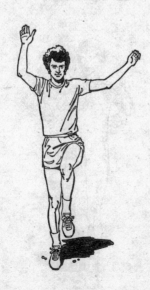

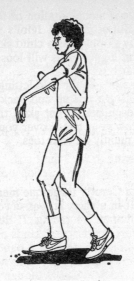

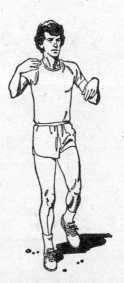

Skip shake-up

This technique is a combination of former Oregon Olympian Dyrol Burleson's and Igloi's warm-up routines. You begin by skipping as a child skips, only raising your knees a bit higher. This will loosen up the legs and elevate the heartbeat.

To shake up, move up the field letting your muscles hang like a rag doll. Do this up and back a distance of about 100 yards each time. First skip, then shake up. Every so often throw your hands over your head and to the sides, but stay mainly on your toes.

Surge

The surge is a Cerutty technique meant to be used at a junction point in a race. It was developed for the crucial parts of competitive racing. It utilizes imagery and technique. There are different kinds of imagery you can use. You can imagine yourself a panther preparing a strike. Or you can imagine that you have the power to pull your opponent back to you as though you were con-

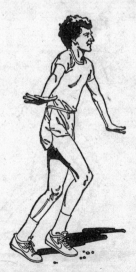

Surge—setting up

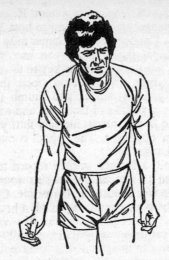

Surge—close up of finger pinching

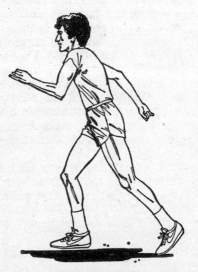

Surge—execution

trolling his movements with a string. You might use it when you're approaching an opponent. Roger Bannister tells of using imagery when closing to beat John Landy in their famous Commonwealth Games mile in 1954.

Regardless of the imagery you use, your hands, now carried at your sides, are the key to the physical exertion of the surge. You should open them to full stretch. Press your forefinger and thumb together, as if they were a gas pedal and the floor, and while making a "ping" sound in the throat, literally hurl yourself forward past your opponent. The "ping" is much like the shout used in karate.

Peter Snell, a former world's record mile runner, reportedly used this technique, minus sound and imagery, when he was running in his prime. Cerutty went so far as to advise his runners to make a head sway immediately after passing the opponent. The reason is that after the surprise wears off, you are susceptible to counterattack.

The surge may strike you as being overly competitive, an act of bad sportsmanship. Actually, the opportunity to use the surge in racing situations doesn't occur that frequently. On the other hand, as a way of raising the heartbeat and deepening oxygen consumption and playfulness, it is unsurpassed. The surge is best practiced off a fresh swing tempo. Do three-quarters of your 100 yards at fresh swing and at the junction point spread the arms slightly, stretch the hands, turn the wrists upward, press the thumb between the front of the forefinger and the knuckle, make a "ping" sound in the throat, and drive forward accelerating up to a good swing at the end.

One tendency to avoid when you are learning the surge is raising your arms too far from your body, so that they become, in effect, flaps that hold the body back. The motions should flow. There should be no jerkiness or loss of forward momentum.

Sprint Form Process

You may not be able to alter your basic, genetically endowed speed, but you can improve it with proper technique. This brings us to the sprint form process, which I learned about from Lee Evans, who still holds the 440-meter world's record at 43.9 seconds and worked with the Esalen Sports Center in 1974. At the time Lee, Ben Tucker, the first American black to run the equivalent of a sub-four-minute mile, and I coached a youth track team sponsored by the local Zen center. This experience helped familiarize me with a number of sprint techniques. Lee and Ben's coach at San Jose College, Bud Winters, teaches sprinters to discipline their bodies through the use of sprint form process. Lee, now the national Olympic coach of Nigeria, is no doubt using this secret with his international class mile relay team.

The key to improving your sprinting ability is increasing your stride length without slowing down the frequency of your steps. You increase stride length by extending your foreleg as far out in front of the body as possible when lifting your knees. You want to maintain a slight forward lean, and stay tall on your toes.

Doing the Sprint Form Process

The sprint form process is best learned in stages, starting with knee action, then leg reach, then arm action and other embellishments.

1. Begin by running in place with your knees high, and run this way down a field or road about 30 yards.

2. Repeat, but when you run your 30 yards, step out as far as possible. Try to get a longer stride without sacrificing leg speed.

3. Bring your arms into play. Arm motion is critical in sprinting. The faster your arms move, the faster you can run. The correct arm movement in sprinting is a parallel motion, but if you watch runners who are tired, you'll frequently see the arms swing across the

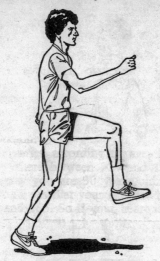

Sprint form—high knees

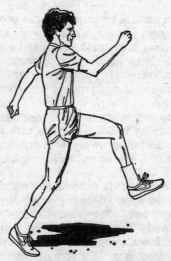

Sprint form—high knees and full leg reach

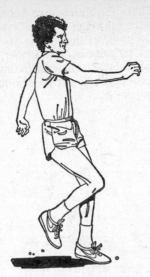

Sprint form—arm action

body. This is a natural tendency (you're protecting the body from fatigue) but it inhibits forward motion. The correct arm action is to reach your hand out as if you were about to shake hands with someone. Then you imagine a vacuum of air pulling your arm back. Lee Evans spent much time in front of a mirror perfecting his arm technique.

To add the arm action to the developing sprint process, begin again by running in place with high knees, and move into the full leg swing, with arm action added. Do the 30 yards a few times, walking back after each run.

4. You're now ready to add a few embellishments. Run tall on your toes, imagining yourself extended 6 inches over your head. Say positive things to yourself like "Loose" and "Free," letting your facial muscles hang on your jowls. You can even experiment with chanting. Lee used to make a sort of "cho-cho" sound through his teeth when he was really smoking.

Once you have the entire form down, practice it a few times. First run through a few 30-yarders, synthesizing the whole process; then three 100-yarders with the sprint form techniques. Remember, this process functions best when lactic acid is inhibiting forward momentum, so its benefits will not be obvious in the form in which you practice it.

Power Run

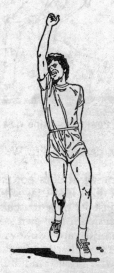

Power run—front view

The power run is a resistance exercise: a run done with a degree of deliberation and strength quite out of proportion to the speed resulting from its practice. Cerutty explained power running in his 1959 pamphlet, *Running with Cerutty.* "In power running we move over the ground at relatively slow speeds, concentrating upon the strength and violence of the movements done. We work our arms and shoulders as vigorously as possible.

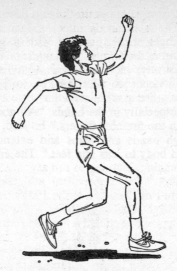

Power run—side view

We exaggerate the degree of lift. We stretch and yearn to be up."

In power running, it does not matter how far you go. The important thing is to exaggerate the lift by placing the body against its own musculature. This is dynamic isometric tension for its own sake. At first, do the power run for just 30 yards, followed by 30 yards of fresh swing. And remember to concentrate. If these exercises are done with intense mindfulness they can increase your strength. After these explosive runs, your regular running will seem easier.

Naturalistic Running

It was always Cerutty's feeling that when your leg and arm variation are synchronized with your breath, the result resembles the asymmetrical striding of a galloping horse. This should be your goal—naturalistic running progressing the way an animal's gait does through parts, each part designed to flow into the next.

In the final stages, you push off the legs during an exhalation that propels the body into a longer stride. This occasional longer stride, coupled with a good swing gait, yields greater distance without additional effort.

Percy Cerutty, of course, was a stylist who believed proper technique was the key to faster, more meaningful running, and believed that style began in the upper body, especially in the hands. "All good running commences in the thumbs, fingers," he said, "and continues through hands and arms and extends through shoulders and body to legs and feet." The end result is naturalistic running: learning to run asymmetrically in a canter or gallop. The prototypical athletes using this technique were Emil Zatopek in the 1950s, Herb Elliott in the '60s, and the Canadian Bruce Kidd, but naturalistic running has not remained a force in running circles. Even so, Cerutty was ahead of the game in observing that "without variation in the upper body we have uniform, uninspiring, mechanical, running action." He foresaw the jogging craze as "negative insanity."

If we follow Cerutty's classical pattern, naturalistic running has five parts: stretch-up, amble, trot, canter, and gallop. Naturalistic running can be applied as a special technique beginning with the trot that starts off on a good swing tempo.

Naturalistic Stretch-up

To familiarize yourself with this approach look at the illustrations and follow the wording. Begin with the stretch-up. "All animals stretch before they run," Cerutty reminds us. Throw your arms over your head while raising up on your toes, and exhale. Do this a few times in a stationary position; then let the arms drop to the sides without any conscious attention to the breath. You are now ready to do the amble.

Naturalistic Amble

When you amble your arms come up alongside the body, as in the tidal breath, but you throw them forward

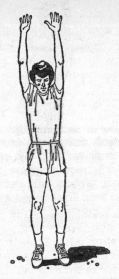

Naturalistic running—stretch-up

on the exhale. Practice putting these two parts together. Stretch up and exhale, letting the arms drop to the sides (on an inhale). Exhale, throwing the arms forward and letting the palms face to the outside. The amble loosens the shoulders and upper carriage.

Cerutty believed that running with a locked elbow joint diminishes the possibility for creative running. Ambling "breaks" the elbow. Practice the stretch-up and amble a few times. You should be standing still on the stretch-up and moving fairly slowly on the amble.

Naturalistic Trot

Actual running begins in the trot, which is the transition into the faster canter and gallop. You begin the trot with an exhale. Then your arms should come up as in the tidal breath or amble, but only to a small distance above the waist. Your exhale should be more of a

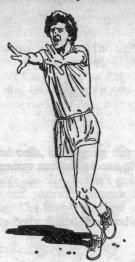

Naturalistic running—amble

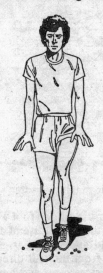

Naturalistic running—exhale during trot

sigh than an energetic breath. Your strides remain of equal length.

The trot shouldn't be done for a long period of time. Its purpose is to set up a rhythm for the faster gaits. To practice the sequence you have learned so far, begin with the stretch-up, proceed into the amble and then fresh swing, using the trot on various, spontaneous occasions.

Naturalistic Canter

When you use the canter technique during a run, you bound forward. The canter step is longer than the

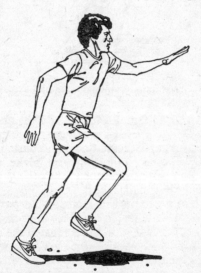

Naturalistic running—canter, side view

other strides. You thrust off one foot with the help of an exhalation and with the proper use of arms and hands.

Choose the lead and follow arms. Either order is OK. Practice going from the trot directly into the canter first, adding the stretch-up and amble later. Exhale as you normally do when trotting, but then, as you take

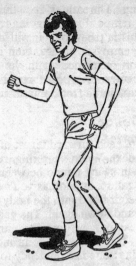

Naturalistic running—canter, hand action

air into the lungs, fill the diaphragm and the chest, lifting the shoulders to get in as much oxygen as possible. Throw your lead arm out and down and during the exhalation let the other, following arm make a much smaller out and down movement, breathing normally to keep your body in balance.

There is a way you can increase the power you gather and release in a canter, using the arms and hands. As Cerutty writes, "When the air is inhaled the drive or pressure initiated by the arms will be 'off,' and when the air is exhaled the drive of the arms will be 'on.'" This is the drive-rest cycle. The same principle applies to the hands. "Only when the fingers are well pinched on or clenched," says Cerutty, "can the full power of the runner be exerted." To relax, you open your hands.

Let's review. The shoulders come up taking in air. On the exhale, the lead arm is thrown out and you thrust off the opposite foot. Your hands should be tight as you initiate the drive on the way up, and opened for relaxation as your hand reaches outward and downward. Don't jump. The canter is a fluid variation of your good swing tempo. Practice going from the trot into the canter. This is the way you will usually use this gait, exhaling to empty the lungs, then using a full inhale and variation of movement in the arms to thrust forward into a canter. Now, go through the whole sequence: stretch-up, amble, trot, and canter.

Naturalistic Gallop

In the gallop, each forward thrust of your lead arm follows into the next. When cantering, remember, your arms are carried in swing tempo between thrusts of the lead arm. In the gallop, as soon as you've exhaled completely you let the air flood into the body and you thrust the lead arm out and down again. The gallop is a powerful motion, so it can only be done for a limited time.

There are two mistakes made in most attempts at naturalistic running: one is a tendency to jump, and the other is failing to bring the follow arm into play to retain balance while moving into the next stride.

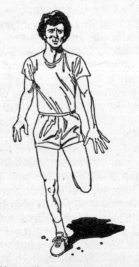

Naturalistic running—gallop

Percy Cerutty sometimes talked of the day when a miler would step up to the start, and beginning with the stretch-up, move into the canter and finally gallop the final yards. According to one calculation, the distance gained in the canter would change a 3:54 mile effort into a 3:47. No wonder Cerutty felt that a 3:40 mile could become common. The only problem is that for most adults it requires a repatterning of mind-body connections to use naturalistic running as a means of going faster.

But let's forget sub-four-minute miles for the moment. The advantage of naturalistic running for the average runner is the sheer fun of it. Try it for yourself. Try breaking out of a long run into a trot or canter. Experiment. Put a trot and a canter into a good swing interval. Occasionally, to loosen the body, go through the whole sequence. When you get in the doldrums remember the canter and gallop. In this way you will escape Cerutty's favorite refrain, "come alive, you hopeless bastard, or better you were dead."

Now that you know a little bit about the different kinds of running, you're ready to see how these different styles fit into these principal approaches in our training program.

Long Continuous Distance

Long continuous distance training was developed by Arthur Lydiard, who has added much to our understanding of how to build endurance into the body. Part of Lydiard's theory is that though speed is inherent, endurance training can increase the ability to maintain basic speed longer. LCD is excellent for this purpose: it increases the ability to develop your maximum oxygen consumption over a long distance.

I recommend nine long continuous distance workouts in the first long-distance training cycle, run in shuffle, fresh swing, or good swing tempo. I have chosen the gait and tempo on my own on the basis of what effort for each particular rank is necessary to bring the heartbeat and the breathing metabolism to a desired level.

If possible, your long continuous runs should be done on a fairly flat surface, beginning from your front door. Run for time rather than distance. If you run for a specific distance, your time for the run usually becomes faster and running faster puts stresses on your aerobic capacity. The best time to run "out" is a few minutes beyond the halfway time. By then you should be well warmed up, and your homeward journey will take less time. When you are doing an LCD workout, keep in mind that you will experience lifeless, listless days. But on such days you have the option of falling back to a shuffle.

The Interval Method

Many running books talk about LCD but go no further. In my view, LCD running is only a part of a complete training program. Just as important is interval training. The interval system I recommend is the one developed by Mihaly Igloi. Your distance will range from 60 to 220 yards; your tempos, from 15 to 80 percent effort. A number of intervals grouped together are called a set.

Intervals are planned runs with specific rest periods. You may run 100 yards, for example, at fresh swing tempo and shuffle 100 yards for recovery. The recovery phase distance should always be the same as that of the interval run. (I have done this for the sake of simplification, so that the workouts can be done without referring to any reference cards.)

Used correctly, interval training improves fitness better than any method I know of. Bill Billinger, whose University of Oregon cross-country team won the 1977 NCAA championship, agrees. "Interval training," he writes, "makes the quickest gains in conditioning."

To get the most out of your interval workouts you'll need a suitable place—a running area you can measure off accurately. A track stadium that has a football field in the middle and grass sections adjacent to the track is ideal. If you don't have this kind of environment available, you'll have to improvise, which you can do in many ways. You can measure the distance between telephone poles, streetlamps, or signs. Even better interval areas are vacant lots or public use grass areas. You can measure off the distances the way a football referee walks off a penalty, one stride to a yard. Get to know the area and become familiar with the terrain.

Our programs include four types of intervals: aerobic, anaerobic, shag, and repetition.

Aerobic Intervals

Aerobic intervals are designed to get the heartbeat into the midpoint of the exercise heart range. (If your pulse range is 134–163, aerobic intervals will get you into the 140–150 range.) For the average runner, this means 100 yards at fresh swing tempo. Aerobic intervals develop your maximum oxygen consumption uptake, and are also thought to increase myoglobin (the oxygen storehouse) in the cells.

Anaerobic Intervals

An anaerobic interval gets the heartbeat to approach and exceed the high point of your exercise heart range. (Using the same range as above, a 30-year-old's pulse range, the range would be 150–190.) As your breathing becomes predominantly anaerobic, your body builds up a lactic acid tolerance and develops the capacity to cope with carbon dioxide tension. You accomplish this with a combination of good swing tempo and sprints.

Shag Intervals

Shag intervals are run when your body has not yet recovered. You might run a 110 yard interval at good swing tempo and follow it by 110 yards at fresh swing. At the end of the second 110 your heartbeat, carbon dioxide tension, and anaerobic debt may still be high but you should begin the next interval anyway. Shag intervals, done properly, improve physical condition quickly.

Repetition Intervals

The repetition runs in any program are 220-yarders, followed by 220 yards of active rest. This distance appears to be most efficient in developing the factors we've been talking about. Use a brisk good swing tempo. The repetition interval is the only interval in which a time is recommended according to individual rank. Remember, most conditioning takes place during recovery. It is during the "rest," whether it be shuffling or walking, that your body is adapting and improving.

Some major coaches argue that a small amount of anaerobic preparation yields all the anaerobic capacity the body can provide. Arthur Lydiard, for instance, argues that "the absolute limit when you are exercising anaerobically is an oxygen debt of 15 liters." He goes on to say that this capacity can be accomplished without any planned program.

This may be true for championship runners who need more pruning of their anaerobic system to have it become operational. But anaerobic running does more than just condition the body to utilize that oxygen debt of 15 liters. It also improves the cardiorespiratory system, the system responsible for bringing oxygen to working tissues and recycling of waste materials. The more efficient the cardiorespiratory system, the quicker the carbon dioxide will be pumped through the lungs; also, the quicker other waste products such as lactic acid are recycled through the liver, the sooner they can reemerge as secondary energy sources.

The Value of Interval Running

Interval training yields a multitude of benefits. It reduces the boredom factor by delivering a wider range of psychological sensations. It makes mental practices easier to handle. Your running area becomes a stage; with intervals, you can choreograph your workouts.

Each interval workout should begin with a warm-up shuffle, followed by a skip-shake-up set. In skip and shake-ups there is no distinguishable rest. Simply turn around and cover the same distance. On some intervals, though, I suggest special techniques like tidal and shoulder breathing, and surging. As for good speed and Cerutty's naturalistic running method, use them at your discretion.

During these intervals you will feel the lungs vary from expansive to moderately relaxed. This is as it should be. The lungs become conditioned to handle various degrees of stress. Like the gills from which they evolved, the lungs thrive on the need to adapt.

Sprinting Intervals

You can use speed to improve your physical condition. Running fast for a short period of time is a highly efficient means of building anaerobic capacity. It brings the heartbeat near its maximum quickly, while increasing the body's oxygen stores. The more you practice running with less oxygen, the easier it becomes to run on a normal supply of oxygen.

But running faster exacts a price. If you run fast for over 15 seconds, you come up against lactic acid accumulation in the muscles. When this hits, your running slows drastically. This is why sprinters must get accustomed to experiencing lactic acid fatigue so that they can handle it in a racing situation.

An Italian fatigue researcher, Rudolfo Margaria, suggests that because there is always a certain period of delay in the onset of lactic acid production even in highly strenuous exercise, you can avoid this production by limiting the activity period to a short time. If you limit spring workouts to short intervals, you will get the benefit of running anaerobically, yet stop before the onset of muscle fatigue. In some of our sprinting we will run 60 yards in a tempo over 85 percent of maximum. You'll rest between each interval so that the heartbeat returns to around 120. The result is a more efficient use of your energy supplies and a rise in the dividing point between aerobic and anaerobic running.

The sprinting program I have outlined does expose you to the end product of anaerobia, lactic acid. The compensating factor will be the improving of your biochemical efficiency.

Do these workouts at the same site as your interval

training. Each workout should include a long warm-up, skip and shake-ups, and the sprint form process. After a few finishing sprints, do the body of the workout. These are 60-yard sprints suggested in the sprinting workouts.

Resistance Running

Resistance running is weight lifting for the legs. The purpose is to build internal power. Resistance running puts grace into your running. You move with more controlled assurance.

This is probably the most underrated and least used of all training methods, but you will notice its effects quickly. Run up a hill or steps and you'll get your heartbeat near its maximum. Your breathing becomes anaerobic almost immediately—so much so that you have to bend over and catch your breath. The magic is that the body almost completely recovers. One second you are exhausted, not able to take another step—then you are ready to run again.

You cannot receive the benefit of resistance running by doing it as part of a long continuous run. It must be done in a suitable environment, as a separate workout. Cement hills are a good environment. So are stadium steps or stairs in an apartment house. Snow or sand dunes are good—even steps of a museum or public building, the way Rocky did it in the movie.

I recommend an uphill environment that takes from 15 to 60 seconds to run. The grade should be steep enough to cause additional strain on your legs and arms, but not so steep that you fall out of a natural stride and end up climbing rather than running. In the Beyond Jogging workshops at the Princess Hotel in the Bahamas we used a beautiful 80-foot sand dune that overlooks the sea. We would visit it and run sets up the dune. This meant up and down a few times, and then rest. Occasionally at the bottom we were out of breath but we hit it anyway. We would go up with sounds in the throat, signifying exhaling as oxygen gushed through our bodies. Our heartbeat would go way up and we quickly accumulated an oxygen debt.

My program uses the simplest form of resistance training: up and down a hill. Arthur Lydiard uses hill training as a separate six-week cycle in his training method. His resistance running is done on a hill that flattens off at the top. He insists that hill training is the most important part of the athlete's training cycles, but for our purposes we will not use resistance running as a distinct phase of the training.

Percy Cerutty emphasized resistance training. Herb Elliott spent long hours on the sand dunes and on the winding uphill trails at the Portsea training camp. When he ran his 3:54.5 world record mile in 1958, he was running only 60 miles a week in training. Much of this was done fast on resistance environments. One great advantage of resistance training is that it gives you a physiological boost without a high risk of injury. In getting the same result from a hard sprint you risk injury to tendons, ligaments, and muscles.

You should run resistance intervals feeling strong and bounding. Be up on the toes; use your arms as leverage. Be well-contained, "up," strong, and dominating. To lose form and tighten going up the hill defeats your purpose. Even when your legs become hard to move and anaerobia sets in, keep your forward momentum. Don't grit your teeth. Abandon yourself to the experience.

Fartlek

You already know a little about fartlek, the method invented in Sweden during the 1940s by coach Gosta Holmer working with athletes Arne Andersson and Gunder Haegg. (*Fartlek* is Swedish for "speed play.") Fartlek means playing with all the gaits, tempos, techniques, and methods we have learned. The Swedes used an up-and-down 2½-mile course through a forest carpeted with pine needles, but you can do fartlek on the same road you do long distance, on an open grass field, a forest path, a golf course, or any other suitable environment.

In fartlek you have the freedom to run at your own discretion. My favorite method is calling the distance. If you are running with a friend you might say, "Let's shuffle to the far tree and fresh swing to a farther signpost." Your friend agrees and the run begins. Then the other partner asks to run fresh swing to a location and then follow with a surge. As an alternative to this socially playful exercise, you can call the distances silently to yourself. When doing fartlek, practice varied options. A good idea is to mentally review your options. If you run slowly (shuffle), increase the tempo a bit and you go into fresh swing, or even faster good swing. Use the breathing techniques described in chapter VI. If you can't do resistance running, do power running. For greater creativity and perhaps new records, experiment with Cerutty's naturalistic running techniques.

VIII

Setting Up Your Own
Six-Week Program

What I've tried to do up to now in this book is
share with you my thoughts, beliefs, and feelings about
running. As you've undoubtedly gathered by now, I
view running as much more than an exercise or a way
of keeping fit.

The programs outlined throughout in this chapter
are designed to help you share some of my feelings and
experiences in running. They are meant to do more than
simply make you a better runner—that is, a runner who
can run longer and faster than before. They are designed
to make the overall running experience a richer, more
enjoyable, more meaningful aspect of your life. These
programs represent an amalgam of training philosophies
that have been given us by some of the world's greatest
coaches and of mental practices that are as ancient as
prayer itself. The ultimate aim of these programs is to
help you bring your mind and body into harmony
through running.

I don't claim categorically that these programs
represent the best system anyone can devise. But one

thing they will do for you is to get you away from joyless and routine "jogging." The schedules and training sequences are based on the most basic physiological principles, and you should be able to notice their effectiveness after your first workout.

The programs are designed to meet your needs regardless of your level of fitness and aspirations in running. The fact that you have no desire to be a running champion doesn't mean that you can't train like one and enjoy the experience of watching yourself become a master of an activity in relation to yourself. You can follow the same schedules followed by world's record holders: the only difference will be in the quantity, quality, and duration of your workouts.

But don't take my word for it. Visit any university that has a good track program. The University of California at Long Beach is one example. The school has many Olympians, among them Dwight Stones and Francie Larrieu. What strikes you when you watch a track workout at this school is how the athletes use the whole area of the training field, how they vary their runs around the field: short and fast, long and slow. In dismal contrast is the way most recreational runners "train": an unvarying, plodding pace around the track. If nothing else, I would like you to take my word that if you allow yourself to follow the variety of programs outlined here, your running performance will improve dramatically, and with this improvement will come a new perspective of yourself both as a runner and as a person.

Some Reflections on Training

Before I get into specifics, let me share with you some thoughts I have about training in general. The entire purpose of training, of course, is to create stresses on the body. It is your body's gradual adaptation to these stresses that results in conditioning. As more and more stress is applied and your body adapts, your capacity for work increases, along with your endurance and stamina.

Given the advanced state of science in this country, you would think that science could tell us which training methods reap the most physiological rewards. Unfortunately, this isn't the case in exercise physiology. Exercise physiologists disagree, for instance, about the relative merits of slow long-distance running as opposed to interval running. And no one has come up with a universally accepted ratio of aerobic to anaerobic training.

I haven't ignored these conflicts in putting together this program but I haven't allowed them to overly inhibit me.

A Special Word to Beginners

If you're a beginner, the best advice I can give is to take the long view. Let the first two weeks be your foundation. Don't expect miracles. Accept the fact that you'll have your days of soreness, of boredom, and of fatigue, but you will also experience days of calm satisfaction. In running the only constant is change. What you experience in the first weeks is a microcosm of how it will be.

Above all, you have to develop mental strength. Do the sequence in your own terms, in your own chosen environments, according to your own running tempos. If someone zooms by you seemingly relaxed and carefree, don't get discouraged and disillusioned. Hold firm to the notion that your running campaign is an exploration of mind and body—a campaign whose aim is to bring heart, breath, and mind into identity. Don't be just another foot in the crowd.

Expect unfamiliar, even peculiar feelings. New approaches can't help but produce them. Remember, you'll be working out in a manner noticeably different from other recreational runners. If these feelings bother you, plan a visit to your local high-school or college track or cross-country team. Get comfortable with the terms for the various methods presented in this book. Watch the team workout and start a dialogue with the coach. Find out more about Cerutty, Igloi, and Lydiard. In short, be an intelligent enthusiast.

Be patient. If you follow the training sequences, physical improvement will happen of its own accord. So let your motto be variety and awareness, variety and awareness! As running becomes more popular there is a temptation to fall in with the others. Fight this tendency. There is too much regimentation in life already. Don't arbitrarily join any running group. Fight for your individuality. The power of the mob mentality is contagious. Strive to be yourself, to find yourself in the running.

Be systematic. Outline practical means to reach your goals, which should be more than an improved performance: look for pleasurable experiences as well. Sample goals include losing ten pounds, or having greater assurance in a usually anxiety-filled situation, or turning a friend on to running. Whatever the goal, make it your decision. Analyze your motivation. If you are running only for health, don't be sucked into racing. If you are after the spiritual qualities, be loyal to the quest. If one of your goals is to move from being a purely recreational runner to being a racer, take the decision seriously. Racing is a powerful ritual; don't take it on lightly.

Dealing with Your Own Attitude

It's possible that this program in its initial stages will make you angry. Maybe you've been jogging several miles a day and you're feeling quite smug about it. You may be saying to yourself, "Now this Spino comes along and I feel guilty and unsure. I feel like I have to start all over again."

If you want to miss a day or change the workout, don't feel guilty. You're the only one who can sense your body on a particular day. The intention of following the training sequence will eventually get you on the best path. Remember, in the course of your search you will experience victory and defeat, ecstasy and boredom, joy and heartbreak. You'll also run into physical soreness, time pressure, and lack of support (not to mention derision) from your most loyal mates. Press on; it is all part of becoming a habitual runner.

Runner's Irony

You will know when you are ready to leave the beginners' rank. You will develop runner's irony. Runner's irony is a combination of Murphy's law ("Whatever can go wrong will") and the steadfastness of seeing a situation through to the end. Runner's irony arms you with the knowledge that after a particularly pleasant workout, the next day you will be sore. On these occasions you'll know how to say "If I had known I'd feel this bad I would have had a couple more to drink last night." Turning sarcasm into energy is a sure sign. Once you use your mind to change fatigue into absurdity, discomfort into silliness, failure into resolve, you're no longer a beginning runner. This variety of response means you have become fit enough to smile, smirk, or jeer at the cycles of health and fatigue all runners experience.

Irony finds a way out. It searches for loopholes. It is a surrender to destiny with a small, wry smile. And when you find your own voice of irony, you will notice, for instance, your shoes don't feel quite as new, that your running gear is becoming a reflection of your personality, that specific places and times of day have a special meaning in your life. You've made the leap. You are a runner.

The Beginning Runner's Two-Week Program

If you're a beginner—if you can't run a mile in less than ten minutes—I strongly recommend the following two-week program before you launch into the six-week program. Its purpose is to help make running a more important part of your spirit and your being. You won't become a marathoner overnight, but your fitness will improve and you will begin to experience the confident glowing feeling that is the ultimate reward in running.

The practical object of this two-week schedule is to get you to run a mile without stopping. During this period you should be doing mental exercises as well as the short version of the stretching set. At first the workouts will be explained in general, nonrunning terms. Later we'll introduce the lexicon for easier communication.

Remember, these workouts are a microcosm of what is to follow in the six-week program. From this simple beginning will come your ultimate routine. Everything that comes afterward will be an extension of this initial routine. You'll need a stopwatch. From then on it's a simple matter of picking a day to start. It can be *any* day—not necessarily the beginning of the week.

Day 1

Your goal is to run slowly (you can refer to this run as jogging) for ten minutes. Running around an oval is OK, but it's better to just go out your front door and start running. Jog about five minutes, stop for a second, and begin jogging homeward. If you feel fatigued, walk for a while. The important thing is to keep moving for the entire ten minutes.

Day 2

Go somewhere where you can measure off a distance of 60 yards. (Try to be as accurate as possible.) If there is a football field handy, you can measure the distance by counting the 5-yard markers. If you're on a flat road outside your house, designate beginnings and ends by markers on the sides of the road. You can measure off the distance by walking off steps, like a football referee counting off a penalty. Each full stride equals a yard.

Near or around the circumference of the area jog for about five minutes, walking if necessary. Then try to run the 60 yards at about half the effort required for an all-out sprint. If you've never sprinted, you won't know what half effort is on the first try, but don't worry about it. Just do the best you can. After the run, walk back to the start. Run three of these 60-yarders at what you think is half effort, walking back the 60 yards each time.

After these three intervals, take a five-minute breather. Walk around. Chat with friends. Or be with your own thoughts. Then do three more 60-yarders in exactly the same way, walking back after each one.

You have now completed an interval workout. You may not feel tired or winded, but don't overdo things by running extra intervals. Stick to the program.

Day 3

Your goal is to run for eight minutes in the same environment you jogged on the first day. The difference will be that this time you're going to vary your running speed. Do part of it at the same pace you ran your intervals the second day. At other times, jog or walk as necessary. Set distances to yourself. Say, "I'll run as far as that tree," or "I'll run for 30 seconds at half effort."

Run various segments of the eight minutes at your own discretion of speed and distance. This type of running is, of course, a fartlek or speed-play workout. Run out five minutes in this way, and three minutes homeward.

Day 4

This day should be a day of rest. Do your long or short stretching set, and perhaps a mental practice, but no running. Observe how your body is responding to the running. Are your joints stiff? How do your legs feel? What is going through your mind?

Day 5

Your goal is to improve your ability to run fast. Do this workout where you did your 60-yard intervals. Approximate a 40-yard distance. After a two-minute warm-up and short stretching set, run two 40-yard intervals, with a walk-back rest in between. You have been running your 60-yarders at half effort, so run these 40 yarders at four-fifths or 80 percent of your maximum. Again, it may take you some time to get a feeling for this tempo, but it will come. After the first two, take a breather for a few moments. Then run two more. After another breather, run two more 40-yarders at 80 percent effort, walking back between each one. You will have run six in all, and you'll have completed your first speed-running workout.

Day 6
Do the same workout as the first day—ten minutes of continuous running.

Day 7
Do the interval workout as you did on the second day, 60 yards six times at half effort.

Day 8
Take a full day's rest, again making sure you do the short stretching set, and perhaps a guided fantasy from chapter IV.

Day 9
Do a fartlek workout like the one you did on the third day, but increase the time out from eight to ten minutes.

Day 10
Jog for 15 minutes, walking when necessary.

Day 11
Do an interval workout similar to the earlier ones but with more volume. Warm up with the customary five minutes of shuffling and then run 60 yards five times at half effort, walking back after each run. Rest five minutes and again run five 60-yarders at half effort. So instead of one set of six runs, you'll be doing two sets of five intervals.

Day 12
Run a ten-minute fartlek workout, just as you did on the ninth day.

Day 13
Have an active stretching and meditation day, but do no running.

Day 14
You are now prepared to run your first mile. Go to a standard track oval (440 yards to each lap) or else measure a mile in a park or on a flat road with your

automobile odometer. To warm up, jog slowly for five minutes. Follow the warm-up with the short version of the stretching set. Now you're ready to run. When you start out on the mile, begin slower than you have been running your intervals. Try to run the entire distance near your maximum, but don't start out too quickly. Time yourself on your stopwatch, or have a friend help out.

If your time is over ten minutes, start the six-week program at the beginner level. If it is between seven and ten minutes, begin at the intermediate level. If you ran in less than seven minutes, contact your local Olympic office.

The Six-Week Program

Training for the sake of training is admirable in the philosophical sense but pointless from a practical point of view. You should always train with specific goals in mind. Experienced runners train for one of four distances: ultralong, long, middle, and sprints.

Each of the programs that follow is geared to one of these four distances. Each program, moreover, is presented in a six-week cycle, and is geared for the special physiological requirements of that distance.

The Sequence

The first six weeks of the program are designed to develop your long-distance running ability. From this base, you should be able to move into either ultralong distances—the marathon—or middle distances—the mile run. The sprinting program, of course, is separate.

Getting Started

Before you get started on your six-week program, you will have to establish your level. We'll be working with five levels:
  • Beginner
  • Intermediate

- Advanced
- Exceptional
- Competitive

A beginner is a runner who has done little or no running; and for runners who fall into this category there is a special two-week program that should precede the six-week program. If you've been running for three times a week and if you can run a mile without stopping in ten minutes or less, you shouldn't consider yourself a beginner.

Establishing Your Level

You can establish your level by taking the first of what we'll be referring to as time assessment runs. Such a run is nothing more than a 1-mile run on a track oval, or on an odometer-measured flat road.

Preparation: Prepare for your mile assessment by shuffling for five minutes and by doing four 80-yard skip-shake-ups. At home beforehand, or directly after the shake-ups, do the shortened version of the stretching set. Follow this with three 80-yards at fresh swing, walking back as the interval rest. Now you're ready to begin the mile at fresh or good swing tempo.

The Run: Although it may be hard for you to assess your amount of effort (if you've never done it before), try to run the distance at about 90 percent of maximum. Time yourself.

Setting Your Level: The following times will designate your rank:

Beginner: 10–15 minutes.
Intermediate: 7–10 minutes.
Advanced: 5½–7 minutes.
Exceptional: 4:40 to 5:30.
Competitive: Anything under 4:40 or its equivalent (9:50 for 2 miles, 15 minutes for 3 miles, 35 minutes for 6 miles, or a 2:50:00 marathon).

Goals

Now that you've established where you stand as a runner, it's time to start setting some goals.

If you're a beginner, your six-week goal should be to run (and walk, if necessary) 3 miles. Your time, at this stage, is not important.

If you're an intermediate, your goal should be to improve your time for a 3-mile run. (I'll talk about establishing your beginning time in a moment.)

If you're an advanced runner, your six-week goal should be to improve your time at 5 miles.

If you're an exceptional runner, your six-week goal should be to improve your time at 7 miles.

And if you're a competitive runner, your goal should be to improve your time at 10 miles.

Setting Time/Distance Goals

You know your level and your general goal. The next thing to do is to run and time yourself at your "goal distance." For example, if you ran a 6:50 mile (advanced), try to run 5 miles (walking, if necessary). Time yourself and use this time as a base on which to measure your improvement after six weeks.

Setting Up Your Workout Schedule

The key to setting up a workout tailored specifically to your goals is metabolic ratio—that is, the ratio of aerobic running to anaerobic running. Here are the recommended ratios.

The Mile: 50 percent aerobic and 50 percent anaerobic.

Long-Distance Running: 65 percent aerobic and 35 percent anaerobic.

Marathon: 80 percent aerobic and 20 percent anaerobic.

If you take the sum of the workouts you do during your six weeks of training, the balance should come out to the above ratios. Try to stick to the ratios, and even if you feel good at the end of a workout, resist the temptation to do "just one more interval." Overtraining can not only throw you off your sequence, it can hurt your body.

Training Methods

Regardless of where you are as a runner and what your goals are, your training workouts should consist of the following methods, although the way in which you schedule and sequence these methods may vary according to your situation.

Long Continuous Running (*LCD*): About 30 percent of your workouts.

Interval: About 25 percent of your workouts.

Resistance: About 10 percent of your workouts.

Speed: About 10 percent of your workouts.

Fartlek: About 20 percent of your workouts.

Time assessments: 5 percent of your workouts.

Another variation in these workouts will be the degree to which you are running aerobically and anaerobically, but we'll get to that point when we talk about specific training regimens.

Time Assessments

The purpose of time assessments is to get your body to go naturally through the entire metabolic process, from aerobic to anaerobic, while moving with an intense heartbeat over an extended period of time. Time assessments are test runs: they accomplish what a race accomplishes but without the haphazard elements of racing. In a time assessment, you go through fresh swing, good swing, tidal breathing, surging, and even cantering and mental practice. Time assessments cannot be done, however, with intervals, because of the rest periods, or long continuous running, where you stick one in gear. But Cerutty set up time assessments through bramble bush circuits. And when Elliott beat everyone's time by 45 seconds on the Hall circuit he and Cerutty both knew he was ready for a new world's record.

Your time assessment in the long-distance program will be half the distance of your preassessment: 1.5, 2.5, 3.5, or 5 miles. Do this on a flat, measured-off road or a standard track oval. And when doing a time assessment always precede it with a short version of the stretching set, and the running warm-up of an interval workout. Either wear a wrist stopwatch or have a friend time you.

Goal Days

Goal days are special time assessments. On goal day you finish up a particular sequence, i.e., six weeks of long-distance training. Warm up as you would for a time assessment or race.

Long Continuous Distance Workouts

There are two types of LCD workouts: LCD (1) workouts, in which you are running between 70 and 85 percent of your exercise heart range; and LCD (2), in which you are running below these percents of your range.

LCD (1)

Beginner
Walk/shuffle/fresh swing (walk when necessary): 20 minutes.
Intermediate
Fresh swing: 30 minutes.
Advanced
Fresh/good swing: 40 minutes.
Exceptional
Good swing: 50 minutes.
Competitive
Good swing: 1 hour.

LCD (2)

Beginner
Shuffle/walk (if necessary): 30 minutes.
Intermediate
Shuffle/fresh swing: 40 minutes.
Advanced
Fresh swing: 50 minutes.

Exceptional
    Fresh/good swing: 60 minutes.
Competitive
    Fresh/good swing: 70 minutes.

Interval Workouts

Beginner
    Shuffle: 5 minutes.
    80 yards skip and shake-ups: 4 times.
    80 yards fresh swing: 6 times, becoming 8 times in 4th week and continuing through end of 6-week cycle.
    Shuffle: 2 minutes.
    Do the following set twice:
    100 yards (50 fresh swing/50 good swing with tidal or shoulder breath at junction point): 2 times.
    Finish with:
    80 yards shake-ups: 4 times.
Intermediate
    Shuffle: 5 minutes.
    80 yards skip and shake-ups: 4 times.
    100 yards fresh swing: 8 times becoming 10 times.
    100 yards good swing in 4th week and continuing on through end of 6-week cycle.
    Shuffle: 2 minutes.
    Do the following set three times:
    120 yards (60 fresh swing/60 good swing with tidal or shoulder breath at junction point): 2 times.
    120 yards (100 good swing/20 sprint with surge at junction point): 2 times.
    Finish with:
    80 yards shake-ups: 4 times.
Advanced
    Shuffle/fresh swing: 5 minutes.
    80 yards skip and shake-ups: 4 times.
    120 yards fresh swing: 10 times becoming 12 times.
    120 yards good swing beginning in 4th week and continuing on through end of 6-week cycle.
    Shuffle: 2 minutes.

Do the following set three times:

140 yards (70 fresh swing/70 good swing with tidal or shoulder breath at junction point): 2 times.

160 yards (140 good swing/20 sprint with a surge at junction point): 2 times.

Finish with:

80 yards shake-ups: 4 times.

Competitive

Fresh swing: 5 minutes.

80 yards skip and shake-ups: 4 times.

180 yards fresh swing: 16 times becoming 18 times.

180 yards good swing in 4th week and continuing on through end of 6-week cycle.

Shuffle: 2 minutes.

Do the following set three times:

180 yards (90 fresh swing/90 good swing with tidal or shoulder breath at junction point): 2 times.

180 yards (160 good swing/20 sprint with surge at junction point): 2 times.

Finish with:

80 yards shake-ups: 4 times.

Resistance Workouts

Beginner

Shuffle/walk: 10 minutes.

Resistance exercises: 15 minutes (including rest periods).

Shuffle/walk: 5 minutes.

Intermediate

Shuffle: 10 minutes.

Resistance exercises: 20 minutes (including rest periods).

Shuffle: 5 minutes.

Advanced

Shuffle: 10 minutes.

Resistance exercises: 25 minutes (time including rest periods).

Shuffle: 5 minutes.

Exceptional

Fresh swing: 10 minutes.

Resistance exercise: 30 minutes (including rest periods).

Fresh swing: 5 minutes.

Competitive

Fresh swing: 10 minutes.

Resistance exercise: 45 minutes (including rest periods).

Fresh swing: 5 minutes.

Speed Workouts

Beginner

Shuffle/walk (if necessary): 10 minutes.

80 yards skip and shake-ups: 4 times.

Sprint form process at 30-yard intervals, 80 yards beginning at fresh swing and accelerating up to good swing: 3 times.

60 yards going to about four-fifths effort with at least 2 minutes rest between each: 4 times.

80 yards shake-ups: 4 times.

Intermediate

Shuffle: 10 minutes.

80 yards skip and shake-ups: 4 times.

Sprint form process at 30-yard intervals, 80 yards beginning at fresh swing and accelerating up to good swing: 3 times.

60 yards going to four-fifths effort with at least 2 minutes rest between each and 5 minutes rest between sets: 2 sets of 4 times.

80 yards shake-ups: 4 times.

Advanced

Shuffle/fresh swing: 10 minutes.

80 yards skip and shake-ups: 4 times.

Sprint form process at 30-yard intervals, 80 yards beginning at fresh swing and accelerating up to good swing: 3 times.

60 yards going to four-fifths effort with at least 2 minutes rest between each and 5 minutes rest between sets: 2 sets of 6 times.

80 yards shake-ups: 4 times.
Exceptional
Fresh swing: 10 minutes.
80 yards skip and shake-ups: 4 times.
Sprint form process at 30-yard intervals, 80 yards beginning at fresh swing and accelerating up to good swing: 3 times.
Competitive
Fresh swing: 15 minutes.
80 yards skip and shake-ups: 4 times.
Sprint form process using 30-yard intervals, 80 yards beginning at fresh swing and accelerating up to good swing: 3 times.
60 yards going to four-fifths effort: 2 sets of 12 times with at least 2 minutes rest between each and 5 minutes rest between sets.

Fartlek Workouts

Beginner
15 minutes, calling the distance.
Intermediate
25 minutes, calling the distance.
Advanced
35 minutes, calling the distance.
Exceptional
45 minutes, calling the distance.
Competitive
55 minutes, calling the distance.

Minimum Days
15 minutes LCD (2) or fartlek for every rank.

Time Assessments
Day 28.
Beginner
Complete run of 1.5 miles (you may walk if necessary).
Intermediate
Time at 1.5 miles.
Advanced
Time at 2.5 miles.

Exceptional
    Time at 3.5 miles.
Competitive
    Time at 5 miles.

Goal Days

Day 42.
Beginner
    Complete run of 3 miles (walk if necessary).
Intermediate
    Time at 3 miles.
Advanced
    Time at 5 miles.
Exceptional
    Time at 7 miles.
Competitive
    Time at 10 miles.

Long-Distance Workouts

In long-distance training, the percentages of use for each method and the range of metabolic ratios are as follows:

METHOD	PERCENT USED	PERCENT AEROBIC	ANAEROBIC PERCENT
LCD	30	80–97	3–20
Interval	24.44	30–90	10–70
Resistance	10	20–60	40–80
Speed	10	5–20	80–95
Fartlek	20	At own discretion	
Time assessment	5.56	60–70	30–40

The number of days allotted for each method are long continuous distance, 9; interval, 7; resistance, 3; fartlek, 6; and time assessments, 2. Long continuous distance ranges from 3 to 10 miles. Runs over this distance are termed ultralong. The range from 0.5 mile to 3 miles is middle distance. From 100 yards to 0.5 mile is a sprint. Continue each day toward your goal. If you miss a day of the sequence, start again by picking up the sequence on the next day. If you miss more than five consecutive days you need to start the six-week cycle over again. A major problem will be minor injuries and travel to unfamiliar environments: do as much of your long continuous distance or fartlek workout as time and physical condition permits. At the end of each cycle you will have the aerobic and anaerobic capacity.

Prepare for your mile assessment by shuffling for five minutes and by doing four 80-yard skip and shake-ups. At home beforehand or directly after the shake-ups, do the shortened version of the stretching set. Follow this with three 80-yard sets at fresh swing, walking back as the interval rest. Now you're ready to begin the mile at fresh or good swing tempo. You will need all your concentration to keep up the momentum in the second half of the run. You may find it difficult to assess your amount of effort, but try to run at 90 percent of your maximum.

The times designating your rank are given on page 154.

Program Outline for Long-Distance Six-Week Training Cycle

Before the long-distance cycle use the following five days of preparation (for all but beginners).

Day 1: 1-mile assessment.

Day 2: rest.

Day 3: Goal distance preassessment.

Days 4 and 5: familiarity with gaits, tempos, techniques, and visualization.

After the Long-Distance Training Cycle

1. Recreational Runner

If you are a recreational runner who exercises for health and an occasional race or fun run you can run indefinitely through the six-week long-distance cycle. The only way to change rank is to improve in the mile run. I recommend that you go through the long-dis-

Rest	LCD (1)	Fartlek	Interval	Minimum day	Speed	LCD (2)
1	2	3	4	5	6	7
Rest	Interval	Resistance	Minimum day	Interval	Fartlek	LCD (2)
8	9	10	11	12	13	14
Rest	Speed	LCD (1)	Minimum day	Interval	Resistance	LCD (2)
15	16	17	18	19	20	21
Rest	Interval	LCD (1)	Fartlek	Resistance	Minimum day	Time assessment
22	23	24	25	26	27	28
Rest	LCD (1)	Resistance	Minimum day	Interval	Fartlek	LCD (2)
29	30	31	32	33	34	35
Fartlek	Interval	LCD (1)	Speed	Minimum day	Rest	Goal day
36	37	38	39	40	41	42

tance training cycle twice and then do the mile program, hoping to improve rank. After this initial 18 weeks, take it upon yourself to chose between long distance, miling, and even sprint workouts.

2. The Marathon

In order to qualify for the marathon training you need to run under seven minutes for 1 mile and average under a 9-minute-mile pace on your long-distance goal run. You should go twice through the long-distance training cycle (12 weeks) before embarking on marathon training. The first marathon of the year needs a minimum of 18 weeks of preparation. This is also the rule if you have not run a marathon in a year. After your first marathon and a week of minimum training (according to the marathon schedule), you can run a marathon again in only 12 weeks. The last week of training before a marathon should be cut in half.

3. Miling

Middle distance, miling, can be done any time after the first two long-distance cycles. Occasionally go through the long-distance cycle as many as four times before doing the mile program. For those interested especially in running the mile, go through the mile cycle a number of times. Take a two-week period in which you race middle distances, running minimum LCD (2) or fartlek on the days between.

Middle-Distance Running

In middle-distance running we will stress the mile because, physiologically, it demands the most elegant combination of strength, stamina, and speed. In this knightly distance, aerobic, anaerobic, and speed variables must be in perfect balance. The mile is the distance in which improvement means the most in relation to optimum physical fitness. This is true even though most runners, especially recreational ones, are more interested in the longer distances. This program is simpler than one which might be personally applied by a coach, but what seems simple between athlete and coach on the track may look like hieroglyphics when written down.

The levels of fitness will correspond to those done during your original assessment. If you live in a climate with intermittent weather you may need to wait until suitable weather to do this program. To accomplish some of these workouts a track field is a great benefit.

The workouts are shown on page 167.

The formula for miling is as follows: LCD (1) (4), LCD (2) (3), intervals (7) of these varieties, aerobic, repetitions, and shags; resistance (5), speed (4), fartlek (5), and time assessment (2).

When you train for the mile you'll find that your long continuous runs become a little slower. You will feel more enthusiastic for your faster workouts, and this euphoric feeling will make the long runs seem boring. Remember, it is important to spend the whole time "on your feet" no matter how slow the pace seems. Even if you occasionally fall all the way back into a shuffle, keep your training equilibrium by completing the workouts.

The new workouts in this schedule are repetition intervals, done at the pace which you hope to run the mile. We are working exclusively with 220-yard intervals. As early as the 1930s Gershler and Reindell discovered that runs of 220 yards at near maximum pace filled the heart almost to its maximum. These intervals work best on a track, but can be accomplished on a grass field or measured road. Outside the goal days or time assessments, this is the only time we will time a workout. This can be done with a wrist stopwatch or a helpful friend.

Igloi and Cerutty believed effort rather than time on a particular day determines the effectiveness of a workout. I've placed the 220s in the training sequence so that you will be rested enough to get the proper physiological effect. A good swing after four or five days of hard training is not the good swing of a workout after a day's rest.

The pace for the 220s will be based on your goal time. For example, if you are running between 5:30 and

1	2	3	4	5	6	7
Rest	Interval (aerobic)	Resistance	Fartlek	Minimum day	Speed	LCD (2)
8	**9**	**10**	**11**	**12**	**13**	**14**
Rest	LCD (1)	Resistance	Interval (aerobic)	Minimum day	Internal Rep	LCD (2)
15	**16**	**17**	**18**	**19**	**20**	**21**
Rest	LCD (1)	Interval (repetitions)	Fartlek	Minimum day	Speed	Resistance
22	**23**	**24**	**25**	**26**	**27**	**28**
Rest	LCD (1)	Interval (repetitions)	Fartlek	Speed	Minimum day	Time assessment (880 yards)
29	**30**	**31**	**32**	**33**	**34**	**35**
Rest	Speed	Interval (repetitions)	Resistance	Fartlek	Minimum day	LCD (2)
36	**37**	**38**	**39**	**40**	**41**	**42**
Resistance	LCD (1)	Interval (shags)	Fartlek	Minimum day	Rest	Goal mile

7:00 for the mile we run the 220s at 45 seconds, with a 220-yard shuffle for the rest period. In these 220s, experiment with tidal breathing, shoulder breathing, good speed, and naturalistic running.

The workouts for miling are all the same as in long-distance training.

Interval Workouts

Interval repetitions will be as follows, for third through sixth workouts:

Beginner

5 minutes shuffle/walk if necessary.
4 times on skip and shake-ups.
2 times 220 yards at 85-90 seconds or at good swing.
220 yards shuffle for recovery.
4 times 80 yards shake-ups.

Intermediate

5 minutes shuffle.
4 times 100 yards skip and shake-ups.
4 times 220 yards in 62-68 seconds or at good swing.
220 yards shuffle for recovery.
4 times 100 yards shake-ups.

Advanced

5 minutes shuffle/fresh swing.
4 times 120 yards skip and shake-ups.
6 times 220 yards in 45 seconds or at good swing.
220 yards shuffle for recovery.
4 times 120 yards shake-ups.

Exceptional

10 minutes fresh swing.
4 times 120 yards skip and shake-ups.
10 times 220 yards in 34-37 seconds or at good swing.
220 yards shuffle for recovery.
4 times 120 yards shake-ups.

Competitive

10 minutes fresh swing.
4 times 120 yards skip and shake-ups.

15 times 220 yards in 30-32 seconds or at good swing.
220 yards shuffle for recovery.
4 times 120 yards shake-ups.

Miling Shags

Beginner
 5 minutes shuffle.
 4 times 120 yards skip and shake-ups.
 2 times 440 yards in 110 shags.
 4 times 120 yards shake-ups.
Intermediate
 5 minutes shuffle.
 4 times 120 yards skip and shake-ups.
 2 times (2) 440 yards in 110 shags.
 4 times 120 yards shake-ups.
Advanced
 5 minutes shuffle.
 4 times 120 yards skip and shake-ups.
 2 times (3) 440 yards in 110 shags.
 4 times 120 yards skip and shake-ups.
Exceptional
 5 minutes shuffle.
 4 times 120 yards skip and shake-ups.
 2 times (4) 440 yards in 110 shags.
 4 times 120 yards shake-ups.
Competitive
 5 minutes shuffle.
 4 times 120 yards skip and shake-ups.
 3 times (4) 440 yards in 110 shags.
 4 times 120 yards shake-ups.

Time Assessments
At end of fourth week: 880 yards.
At end of six weeks: 1 mile.

Marathon Schedule

For the marathon schedule the qualification is a seven-minute mile and the ability to run the goal distance under a nine-minute-mile pace.

1	2	3	4	5	6	7
Rest	LCD (1)	I (aerobic)	Resistance	Fartlek	Minimum day	LCD (2)
8	**9**	**10**	**11**	**12**	**13**	**14**
Rest	LCD (1)	I (aerobic)	Fartlek	Resistance	Minimum day	LCD (2)
15	**16**	**17**	**18**	**19**	**20**	**21**
Rest	LCD (1)	Fartlek	I (aerobic)	Resistance	Minimum day	LCD (2)
22	**23**	**24**	**25**	**26**	**27**	**28**
Rest	LCD (1)	I (shags)	Fartlek	Resistance	Minimum day	Time assessment
29	**30**	**31**	**32**	**33**	**34**	**35**
Rest	LCD (1)	Fartlek	Resistance	I (aerobic)	Minimum day	LCD (2)
36	**37**	**38**	**39**	**40**	**41**	**42**
Rest	Resistance (shags)	Resistance (shags)	LCD (1)	Minimum day	Rest	Goal run

The marathon training is broken down into the following workouts: LCD (1) (6), LCD (2) (4), interval (6), fartlek (6), resistance (6), time assessments (2), minimum days (6). The aerobic-anaerobic ratio is approximately 80 percent aerobic to 20 percent anaerobic.

This initial 30-week buildup may seem like a long time, but it is better to be prepared for your first venture than to end up with, literally, a bad taste in your mouth. Be very careful after running your first marathon. Your body will be susceptible to injury. Ron Wayne points out that the most serious injuries often occur after successful marathons. The run feels easy and you want to immediately resume heavy training. Beware!

To be safe, think seriously before running more than three marathons a year. Wayne ran six under 2:20:00 in 1977, but this kind of "Lou Gehrig" strength is very unusual.

Advanced

LCD (1)
50 minutes fresh swing.

I (Aerobic)
5 minutes shuffle.

4 times 120 yards skip and shake-ups.

2 sets of 14 times 120 yards good swing, with approximately 2 minutes shuffling between sets.

4 times 120 yards shake-ups.

Fartlek
40 minutes, calling the distance. It is recommended that in this section you run 2 times 15 minutes at good swing, but again this day of training is at your discretion.

LCD (2)
2 hours shuffle—can be 9-minute or slower pace.

Minimum Day
30 minutes shuffle.

I (Anaerobic)
5 minutes shuffle.

4 times 120 yards skip and shake-ups.

2 times (3) 440 yards in 110 shags.
4 times 120 yards shake-ups.

Resistance

10 minutes shuffle.
25 minutes resistance exercise.
4 minutes shuffle.

Time Assessments

(1) 8 miles at good swing.
(2) 6–12 mile race or 6-mile assessment.

Last week of cycle on race month: half the workouts of LCD (1), shags, and minimum day leading to race.

Excellent category

LCD (1)

1 hour good swing.

I (Aerobic)

5 minutes shuffle.
4 times 120 yards skip and shake-ups.
2 sets of 16 times 140 yards good swing, with approximately 2 minutes of shuffling between sets.
4 times 120 yards shake-ups.

Fartlek

45 minutes, calling the distance. A recommendation is 2 times 20 minutes at good swing, but this workout should be run as you feel with the intervals at your own discretion.

LCD (2)

2:45:00 at shuffle/fresh swing can be a bit under 8-minute pace.

Minimum Day

40 minutes shuffle/fresh swing.

I (Anaerobic)

5 minutes shuffle.
4 times 120 yards skip and shake-ups.
2 times (4) 440 yards in 110 shags.
4 times 120 yards shake-ups.

Resistance

10 minutes shuffle.

30 minutes resistance exercises. (This means you stay at your environment for 30 minutes; run at your own intensity.)

5 minutes shuffle.

Time Assessments

(1) 10 miles at good swing.

(2) 6–12-mile race or 8-mile assessment.

Last week of cycle on race month: half the workouts of LCD (1), shags, and minimum day leading to race.

Prerequisite: Sub-2:40:00–2:27:00 Marathon

LCD (1)

1½ hours fresh swing.

I (Aerobic)

5 minutes shuffle.

4 times 120 yards skip and shake-ups.

2 sets of 16 times 180 yards good swing.

1 lap shuffle.

4 times 220 yards good swing.

4 times 120 yards shake-ups.

Fartlek

1 hour, recommended 2 times 25 minutes good swing, but this workout should be run as you feel with the intervals at your own discretion.

LCD (2)

3 hours at fresh swing at 7:30–8:00 pace.

Minimum Day

1 hour shuffle/fresh swing.

I (Anaerobic)

5 minutes shuffle.

4 times 120 yards skip and shake-ups.

3 times (4) 440 yards shags at 110.

4 times 120 yards shake-ups.

Resistance

10 minutes shuffle.

45 minutes resistance exercises. (This means you stay at your environment for 45 minutes; run at your own intensity.)

Time Assessments

(1) 12 miles at good swing.

(2) 6–12-mile race or 12-mile assessment.

Last week of cycle on race month: half the workouts of LCR (1), shags, and minimum day leading to race.

National and International class Marathon (2:15:00 to 2:27:00)

This constitutes twice-a-day workouts. A sample schedule is shown on pages 175 and 176.

Sprinting

Great sprinters are born, not created. The ability to run fast is genetically bred directly into the muscle fiber. But though there is no substitute for basic sprinting ability, proper training and technique can help, if only to certain limits.

The idea behind sprinting training is to increase your strength, help you relax more, and teach you proper technique. This is why at least two cycles of the miling program are recommended before concentrating on sprinting. This is why I stress the sprint form process. Sprinters will find the relaxation techniques, especially some of the mental rehearsal and autogenic guided fantasies, extremely effective.

Preparing to sprint invariably means getting ready to race. This gets to be a problem for the recreational runner. British-born Olympic 400-meter hurdle gold medalist David Hemery recently pointed out that little is written about sprinting in the popular running magazines. The concept of runner's high is almost always associated with jogging or longish running. Recreational runners are most often not sprinters. For this

	1st week	2nd week	3rd week
Monday	1 — 30 min. minimum distance	8 — 30 min. minimum distance	15 — 30 min. minimum distance
Tuesday	2 — AM: 12 miles fresh swing; PM: 8 miles fresh swing	9 — AM: 12 miles; PM: 8 miles fresh swing	16 — AM: 12 miles; PM: 8 miles fresh swing
Wednesday	3 — 5 min. shuffle, 6x100 shakeup, 2 sets of 16x220 good swing, 8x330 fresh swing, 6x220 good swing	10 — same as above	17 — AM: 1 hr. 15 min. fartlek; PM: 2x35 good swing
Thursday	4 — resistance same as Saturday AM of 2nd week	11 — fartlek same as Wed. of 3rd week	18 — Interval same as Wed. of 1st week
Friday	5 — AM: 1 hr. 30 min.; PM: 2x35 min fartlek; fresh swing; PM: 30 min.	12 — AM: 1 hr.; PM: 30 min. fresh swing	19 — AM: 1 hr.; PM: 30 min. fresh swing
Saturday	6 — AM: 1 hr. 30 min.; PM: 30 min. fresh swing	13 — AM: 10 min. warm, 50 min. resistance 20 min.; PM: 30 min. fresh swing; fresh swing	20 — same as above
Sunday	7 — 22 miles 7-7:30 pace	14 — 7-7:30	21 — 22 miles 7-7:30

	Monday	Tuesday	Wednesday	Thursday	Friday	Saturday	Sunday
4th week	22 30 min. minimum distance	23 AM: 12 miles PM: 8 miles fresh swing	24 5 min. fresh swing 6x100 shakeup 3x6 laps of 220 shags with no shuffle rest	25 fartlek same as Friday of 1st week	26 same as resistance Sat. 2nd week	27 AM: 1 hr. fresh swing PM: 30 min. fresh swing	28 22 miles 7-7:30
5th week	29 30 min. minimum distance	30 AM: 12 miles PM: 8 miles fresh swing	31 fartlek same as Friday 1st week	32 resistance same as Saturday of 2nd week	33 same as Wednesday 1st week Week I aerobic	34 AM: 1 hr. fresh swing PM: 30 min. fresh swing	35 22 miles 7-7:30
6th week	36 fartlek same as Friday 1st week	37 resistance Saturday 2nd week	38 shags same as Wednesday of 4th week	39 AM: 12 miles fresh swing PM: 8 miles fresh swing	40 AM: 1 hr. fresh swing PM: 30 min. fresh swing	41 30 min. fresh swing	42 Race 3-12 miles

reason, I do not provide a complete training guide, but rather an outline and suggestions.

You can notice a sprinter because they walk as slow as they run fast. They will be the last to get off a team bus, and the slowest getting to any team function. But when they go, watch out!

The Practice of Sprinting

If you wish to be a proficient sprinter you need to do more than the 60-yarders of this book. This is because sprinting challenges the regulatory systems to a greater extent. The degree to which you become anaerobic, and the acidity level of the blood, is proportionately higher in hard sprinting. As mentioned in the section on methods, it takes 12 to 15 seconds for lactic acid to build up. The 60-yarders let you work under anaerobic conditions without lactic acid buildup. Longer runs tax the physiology to a much greater extent. And as in all things, your body must practice what it hopes to accomplish.

Sprinting is based on quality, not quantity. Some outstanding sprinters do as little as three to five intervals in a workout. These, though, are done quickly, usually a bit under and over the planned assessment distance.

Proper form and an aerobic buildup program do help, but not as much as raw ability. Sprinters are usually mesomorphs, muscular types whose bodies can withstand the pressures exerted upon the speeding body. Still, you may want to dabble in sprinting as a recreational diversion from the "plodding" of long-distance running.

The environments for good sprint training are the running track, an uphill and a level road, or park area. Use the track for repetition-type speed intervals, the incline for building anaerobic reserves and leg strength, and the roads for the necessary aerobic running that keeps up the endurance base.

Championship sprinters train the year round. The fall is the season for strength work, by running hills and weight training, also aerobic base conditioning. A modern program emphasizes proper technique, biomechanical evaluation, and breathing as well as mental and relaxation practice. Winter can mean racing indoors under or above the goal distances. This leads to a program that peaks in late spring and summer. If you're a recreational runner interested in improving your ability to run fast, do mile training in the fall, and use the kind of midseason training I will outline, that moves into peaking in the late spring and summer.

Sprint Technique

You must maintain strength and flexibility throughout the year, so as a sprinter you should do the stretching aspects outlined in this book. Perfecting your sprint form is invaluable. The velocity of force in running fast attempts to throw you into accessory movements, and a relaxed body that moves in disciplined form will handle fatigue with more ease. Percy Cerutty's idea of opening the hands on the exhale and drive and gripping the hands for the drive forward is also very helpful.

Sprinters' Training Sequences

The basic principle of sprint training is to run *under* distance a number of times and *over* distance a few times. To do this, we employ the three methods of aerobic running, resistance running, and interval repetitions. Below are examples of two-week cycles: (1) a sprinter's buildup period which would follow miling training in the fall; (2) the type of training which would be done during the competitive season. If you sprint it will have some competitive aspects, so if this outline leaves you wanting more, refer to Bud Winters, *So You Want to be a Sprinter,* or the work of Jim Bush, the track coach at UCLA. They have produced some of the best sprinters in the world.

This outline is a bit more typical for men running 220 to 330 yards; those training for the 60 or 100 would need to cut down on the repetitions and boost speed.

The sprinter's training cycle might look like this:

	Monday	Tuesday	Wednesday	Thursday	Friday	Saturday	Sunday
1st week	LCD (1)	Resistance	220s	Resistance	Fartlek	Resistance	Intervallike 150s; 220, 330 good swing
	1	2	3	4	5	6	7
2nd week	Minimum Distance 15 min.	Intervals, over distance, 2 times 600 yards each	Fartlek	Resistance	LCD (2)	Rest	Goal Practice
	8	9	10	11	12	13	14

A racing period schedule for the sprinter could look like this:

	Monday	Tuesday	Wednesday	Thursday	Friday	Saturday	Sunday
1st week	Intervals over distances, 4 times, 330 yards each (1)	Resistance (2)	Intervals, underdistance, 2 times, 660 yards each (3)	Fartlek (4)	110s, etc. (speed) good swing (5)	Rest (6)	Rest (7)
2nd week	Intervals, over distance, 4 times 330 yards each (8)	Resistance (9)	Intervals, underdistance, 2 times, 660 yards each (10)	Fartlek (11)	110s, etc. (speed) (12)	Rest (13)	Rest (14)

If 60 yard intervals, run shorter and faster.

Appendix

A good deal of the material covered in other running books is conspicuously missing from this one. This is not because I consider diet, for example, unimportant, but because I have tried to stress in this book information and material that is new to you. All the same, here are some brief thoughts on some of the basics of running you might be interested in.

Equipment

First things first. Don't buy a new sweat suit. The best clothes are old sweat shirts and last year's swimsuit. Even a new pair of running shoes is not an absolute necessity. Michael Murphy, Esalen's founder, ran in simple sneakers until he had run the mile in under 6:00. Ted Corbitt, the legendary New York City marathoner, ran his early thousands of miles in street shoes.

When you do buy a pair of running shoes, be careful. Don't be deceived by "cosmetic" types. Buy a brand name. Inadequate shoes are the worst investment you can make. Bypass extraheavy shoes designed primarily for cement roads. You want a shoe to work for grass, dirt, uphill—even racing. Ask the dealer for something between a road and a purely racing shoe. Make sure it has some bend to the sole, and feels balanced on your foot. Give yourself enough room to move your toes. Socks? Socks with heels are better than tubes which have a tendency to roam all over your foot. And beware of tight socks. They can cramp your feet as much as tight shoes.

If the weather is moderate, all you need is a singlet and a pair of shorts. For men, athletic supporters are passé. Wear shorts with a built-in support or wear jockey-style underwear. Some runners wear women's underwear for races. Women should wear a bra with enough support to keep the breasts from bouncing.

There are a number of inexpensive wrist stopwatches available in today's running marketplace. They are indispensable: They will enable you to monitor your own workouts.

Environments

Except for long continuous running and resistance exercises, try to avoid hard surfaces. Cerutty used to say that athletes who train mostly on hard surfaces are "noted for short strides and mincing gaits." Hard surfaces are hard on your lower back, ankles, and knees.

The best environment is the most accessible one. A beautiful trail around a deserted lake is ideal, but not if it's a 30-minute drive away. Don't overlook the obvious. Industrial parks in the inner city sometimes have long, open, infrequently traveled roads.

Weather

If you are prepared, you can run in any weather without too many problems. If it's cold, several layers are a better buffer against heat loss than one bulky set. Wear a cap and gloves. Long-john underwear will keep you warm and give you freedom of movement. You can run in a snowstorm with gloves, cap, long johns, undershorts, and a hooded sweat shirt. Don't worry about the cold. It won't damage your lungs. Practicing Stough's breathing coordination will help your lungs acclimate.

Hot weather is trickier. The big danger is that you can get dehydrated without realizing it. Running in hot weather is especially dangerous when the temperature and humidity are both high. Remember to drink liquids; ones with electrolytes like ERG, Bodypunch, or the commercial Gatorade replace lost minerals. Wear light-colored, lightweight tops. Better, go topless. Don't get yourself sprayed with water. Instead of cooling the body, it will only keep the heat in without letting the skin breathe.

Wind? Bless it. It gives you a natural resistance workout. Herb Elliott ran on the wind-torn beaches of Australia, struggling in unison with nature. City smog, on the other hand, is bad news. If you live in a place where smog alerts are announced, run only early in the morning or late in the evening. Smog was the only reason Igloi ever canceled or shortened a workout.

Food

A runner's body operates most efficiently on carbohydrates and fats. For this reason, the ideal runner's food is a lactovegetarian diet. Percy Cerutty was a pioneer in the application of nutrition to running. "All the training is useless," he once wrote, "if the engine is not stocked or fed upon the best fuel (food) possible to obtain, and adequately in quantity."

What are some of the foods Cerutty recommends for the runner? A scan of Cerutty's Portsea training camp's menu tells the story: fruits, vegetables, nuts, eggs, cheese, lightly cooked meats, fish, and poultry, peanut butter, honey, jams, potatoes, beans, thick soups.

Stick to this kind of food and stay away from the obvious hazards like sugar, cigarettes, alcohol, and excessive red meats.

And what about runners who need to lose weight? Running and aerobic fitness are directly correlated with weight. The thinner you are, the easier it is to run and gain aerobic fitness. Being overweight means you have to work harder to achieve the same physiological benefits as somebody who isn't overweight. But running won't help you lose weight unless you are eating properly too.

How do you go about losing weight? Given the number of books on the subject, I could hardly expect to cover the subject in a page or two. I'll say this, though: if you follow the training sequences, and cut back 200 calories a day, you can lose weight. Buy a bathroom scale and weigh yourself daily. Aim at losing one pound a week. (Anything more is water loss that will easily return.) Each morning check the scale. If after a week you haven't lost a pound, cut back on your intake. This is not as easy as it sounds. Percy Cerutty placed high value on conquering "belly hunger." Don't expect the weight to come off right away. Exercise physiologist Laurence Morehouse points out: "If you're overweight and underexercised when you start your program, you may not lose weight for a while, because as you build muscle, bone and blood, the weight of those vital tissues may disguise the loss of fat." If you are faithful to the running, and careful about what you eat, excess weight will disappear.

Mental practice can help. Sylvia, a woman in a long-term (6-month) program conducted in our Esalen Sports Center in 1976, realized during body image meditation that she had always sought weight loss to please others. When she changed her attitude to one in which she sought to lose weight for her own feelings of health and well-being, 15 pounds vanished seemingly overnight.

Vitamins

Some runners take dozens of vitamin pills a day. Others see them as worthless. I recommend them, but not in excess. The best vitamins for runners are B complex for oxidation, C to fight odd colds, and E for endurance. Replacing the trace minerals magnesium and potassium is important too. Vitamins are best taken in concentrated time periods. Take them for three or four months in a row and then rest a month. This practice is a safeguard against immunity and adaptation.

Illness and Injuries

I am not a physician but I might be able to offer insights and suggestions from information gathered through the running community, the body-oriented human potential movement, and my personal experience. The best overall advice about running injuries that I know was given by former *Runner's World* editor Joe Henderson: "If the pain goes away when you begin running, keep going. If it persists, or gets worse, stop."

Trust your body. The ability of the body to adjust itself and eventually eliminate an injury or pain is amazing. Most runners have experienced annoying injuries that suddenly disappeared.

Not that you should become unconscious of your physical state. If you have any doubt about the functioning of your heart or lungs, for instance, deal with it immediately. Visit your family doctor or a specialist. Get an EKG test. This will provide you with a diagram of your heart rhythm. Don't be a hypochondriac, but check yourself regularly for signs of fatigue. George Sheehan recommends taking a daily fitness index: "When you wake in the morning, lie in bed for five minutes, then take your pulse. Also check your weight and breathing." Be alert to any sudden variance. If you have serious doubts, get a full medical checkup.

The local podiatrist has become a local hero for many runners. Podiatrists contend that weakness or structural problems in the foot greatly affect the rest of the body. They insist that if you are off kilter even slightly, you'll eventually develop foot, leg, and back problems. Realign the body, correct the imbalance, and allow the body to heal.

Arch appliances designed by podiatrists have helped thousands of runners, but there are other alternatives. Just as the body can be balanced from the feet upward, it can be aligned from other perspectives.

The feet are only the focal point. The real problem is the way gravity affects the body, and there are a number of practitioners who physically manipulate the body to place it on the correct alignment, including chiropractors, osteopaths, and rolfers. The chiropractor realigns the verterbrae of the spinal column to release pinched nerves. Osteopaths are medical doctors who specialize in the relationship between muscles and bones. Rolfers, through deep massage, manipulate the muscle connecting tissue. This realigns the various sections of the body so that they work in harmony.

There are many other possibilities of reducing pain or dealing with injury, including acupressure and acupuncture, various forms of massage, and psychophysical disciplines such as bioenergetics. The mental practices in chapter VI and the stretching sets can help enormously in preventing injuries. The breathing exercises can help you feel calm and relaxed. I haven't mentioned injuries like muscle pulls and twisted ankles, which call for traditional athletic training care.

Weight Lifting

The top coaches disagree on the value of weight training for runners. Arthur Lydiard feels that since arms are only for balance, weight lifting is superfluous. Igloi would even brag about his athletes' weakness, pointing out that one of his runners, Iharos, couldn't lift a chair over his head when he was the world's best distance runner.

Cerutty was different. He was a pioneer in weight training. He suggested five basic lifts—one-arm swing, curls, press, dead lift, and bench press—to be done a few times with heavy weights so as to build strength. He felt that weight lifting was essential for competitive middle-distance runners and sprinters, but less important for recreational runners and for runs over 3 miles, where it is more important for a runner to be flexible and aware than strong.

Running Partners

When you run well with a partner, a kind of bio-entertainment occurs. Your stride, breath rhythms, and perhaps even heartbeats become synchronized. Author George Leonard describes these "crystalline moments" in his book *The Silent Pulse*. Some of the best relationships develop when an experienced runner takes a younger runner under his wing. In other situations, you should exercise great care. Be leery of partners who profess noncompetitiveness and then rush you through your stretching routine, or else continually want to change the workouts. A training partner doesn't have to be entirely selfless, but you don't want to become someone else's sparring partner.

I've had only three running partners: Martin Miller at Syracuse University, Bob Deines in the San Francisco Bay Area in the 1960s, and Michael Murphy with Esalen in the '70s. What all these men had in common was a quick wit, a sense of the absurd, and a deep love for the natural act of running. Physically we complemented each other's training needs. I had more speed than Martin Miller, for example, but he could go for miles. Bob Deines taught me how to run long distance. Michael Murphy was the first athlete I ever coached.

In one recent race I experienced the positive and negative aspects of a randomly chosen running partner. I first fell in with a man who seemed to bump into me on every third or fourth step. A shoulder, a hand, an elbow—nothing intentional. It didn't throw me off my stride but after a few miles I was tight and irritable. Later, an easier-striding young man pulled up. Without effort we seemed to breeze past a few clusters of runners and soon were pulling for each other. Soon we found out we were both born in Margaret Hague Hospital, in New Jersey.

Plateaus

Your physical condition will improve in jumps rather than a straight line. This move frequently comes suddenly, but quite sequentially, and it doesn't require any additional effort. Over a period of months you will experience a cycle. The plateauing at the end of the cycle of fitness doesn't mean that you will be able forever to duplicate a particular time. In your first assessments you will have an experience of your body coming around. These first surges of power will be a memorable occasion, a first love between you and your body. They may even produce peak experiences. Plan for the plateaus and accept the rushes of physical power they provide. It is part of your just rewards.

Spouses and Lovers

It's great if your lover or spouse can also be your running partner, but the relationships often don't mix. Time spent together exercising can create a calm that is a wonderful prelude to lovemaking, but the down side is having to adapt to each other's workouts, and the likelihood of argument. A lot of energy gets released when you run, and things that have been brewing under the surface can rise to the surface. I have even heard of lovers coming to blows between strides. If your mate is on the same level of fitness as you, running together may work out, but don't sacrifice the workouts for the sake of camaraderie. Instead, do the first part of the workout together, and then go your separate ways.

How to Run a Race

Racing is a ritual, a planned escapade in which you strive to reach your maximum physical and mental powers. We get our bodies fit for health, but we race seeking adventure. Racing actually takes away from physical condition. It tears the body down; it's a withdrawal from your fitness bank account. Before a race you will be loose and receptive. You are in the chips. Afterward, you are broke.

If an aerobic workout is fluidity, a race is violence. So prepare as though you were preparing for combat. Good and bad performances needn't be arbitrary. The secret to success is to plan your training. Planning correctly, what Cerutty called "intelligent training," brings you to the race situation at your best.

When you plan your training campaign, be alert to signposts along the way. Notice how easily you accomplish what had once been difficult workouts. Your time assessments will reflect your improvement. If you follow the plans in this book, you will face a race not wondering if you will improve, but how much.

The race should be for self-expression. Through it you may, on occasion, find truth. Cerutty put it best: "Racing is an art form that calls for no less than the full expression of the person—physically, mentally, and spiritually." Racing has all the elements of Zen: deprivation, dedication, one-dimensional zeal. These qualities can deliver ecstasy. But to exult in this glory can mean deceiving yourself.

If you are a beginning runner or one of those just breaking out of the jogging syndrome, you will have it the easiest. You will improve physically as well as develop a new perspective. Runners with racing experience often face an additional dilemma: purpose and motivation. Where is the meaning? In your training you may come upon beautiful experiences. Most likely, though, your real understanding of yourself will come through racing. You must cultivate it if you are to use it as a gateway to greater self-knowledge. So race as a God-seeking artist. Let your anxiety be your stage fright.

Mental Preparation

The best mental preparation is accomplished in the days before the race. Mentally rehearse your perfect scenario. If it is a road race, picture each lap and the energy you will exert. Go over the stages in your mind's eye, and see yourself accomplishing each segment successfully. Your prerace manner should reflect your natural temperament. Don't worry about being psyched out. As a rule, the more relaxed you are, the better you will race. Your body knows what is expected.

Trust it and it will respond. You need to experiment to find out how you relax. Some runners strive on separate solemnness. For others, this causes stress. Find your own way.

Resting

Some runners hardly sleep the night before a race. Many sprinters like to race off that "jangly" feeling you get from lack of sleep. What is important is having your environment the way you want it. Get away from the pressure of the race. At the Olympic Village the busiest place is the discotheque. Ben Jipcho, one of the great professional runners of all time, would sleep for an entire day before a big race, but liked to attend social engagements up to the time the rest period began. Lee Evans likes to wake early on race day and go fishing. Coaches who make you stay up without friends or relatives are not only unreasonable, they are throwing off your relaxation process. Peter Snell set a world's record for the mile on his honeymoon!

If you are troubled by not being able to sleep, try this visualization, which is a bit like counting sheep. See yourself standing in front of a blackboard and writing the number 100 in chalk on the blackboard. Then watch yourself erase the 100 and replace it with a 99, etc., all the way down to 0 if necessary. If you make 0, begin again at 99. Soon you will be asleep.

The Racing Diet

When preparing for a race, stay fairly close to your regular diet. Special foods don't give much of an extra boost unless the race is more than an hour and a half. Arthur Lydiard recommends eating 200 grams of barley sugar in the 36 hours preceding a competition. Physiologist David Costill says a cup of black coffee one hour beforehand will activate the burning of fats earlier in the race. Other coaches suggest fasting up to race time to get that light-headed, cleaned-out feeling.

Cerutty's athletes ate large salads. Lydiard recommends a breakfast of cereals, lightly cooked eggs, and coffee or tea for a morning race. If another meal is needed, make it honey sandwiches or baked beans.

For races over an hour and a half, use the carbohydrate loading system. Run to exhaustion seven days before the race. This depletes the body of most of its carbohydrates. Spend three days eating high-protein foods like cheese and meats, then add on lots of carbohydrates like spaghetti and breads. This will add glycogen to your muscle cells.

Warming Up

You should taper your training so it is easier to warm up for a race than for a regular workout. Even though you are feeling loose, don't neglect the essentials. Do your regular meditation and stretching set before coming to the site of the race. At the track or road, shuffle for 10 to 20 minutes. Do 4 to 10 skip and shake-ups. Follow this by lying on your back and going through the breathing coordination cycle. (Don't forget to stay warm.) Lie down or walk slowly near the starting line until a few minutes before race time. Then do your second warm-up, consisting of a shuffle and a few 80-yard good swings. By now your heartbeat will be slightly elevated (it will be from the excitement of the race, anyway), your muscles and ligaments stretched, and your concentration focused.

Final Preparations

Final details can mean the difference between success and defeat. Don't let the benefits of your training be lost through negligence. Check the time when your race begins and know how to get to the start. A last-minute rush will get you to the line rattled and tight. Be sure your toenails are cut. In long races put vaseline on nipples and groin. In road races know the course, especially if you plan to be running with the leaders. Empty your bowels. You should do this before leaving home because arrangements at race sites are often inadequate.

When you get your number, rip off the paper to the outside of the print so that it doesn't flap in the wind. In cold weather apply a hot rub around the small of the back and legs (tiger balm is good). In hot weather wear a light-colored perforated shirt. Invest in a pair of racing shoes. They will be lighter than normal in weight and design. Double-knot your shoes! You'd be amazed at the countless great races that have been lost through untied shoelaces.

Anything can happen from here on out. It is a coach's job to mentally prepare the athlete to deal with any contingency. But a coach who makes the athlete dependent does him a great disservice. In the throng we must know our identity.

The Start

When standing at the starting line try this visualization. Locate your awareness in your chest and lower back. Take a few breaths into these areas. Do this for a few moments. Just before the start, release your mind from this discipline and give yourself the image of flowing down a river. Begin the race with this image in your mind.

But stay aware. Getting off the line efficiently can mean the difference between a relaxed, self-controlled race and a nervous, anxious one. In some track races you will be given a position, but mostly you will be left to your own discretion. Try to line up to the outside of the group. It is much better to veer in from the side under your own control than to be cut off. Start substantially, without being aggressive. Secure your "space" and give yourself running room. In large-scale road races you may not be able to run right after the starting gun. Don't fight it. The traffic will open up soon enough. Arrive at race pace as soon as possible with the least amount of jostling. A smooth race is usually the fastest.

Racing Attitudes

Different coaches recommend different styles of racing. A basic prototype is the runner who sprints from behind to victory. Cerutty disliked this approach, believing a leader should take responsibility for the race. Igloi was more concerned with times and records. He would give the runner a goal time. Both coaches, however, felt it was more honorable to run to your maximum than to win in slow timings.

Although some champions have used tactics to disrupt their opponents' momentum, the best plan is to run a fairly even pace. Vladimir Kuts, the great Russian champion of the 1950s, would throw in bursts in midrace to confuse his opponents. If they followed, and ran his race, they would wear out.

World's record races have usually been run in the following lap/speed sequence: (1) second fastest, (2) third fastest, (3) fourth fastest, (4) fastest. This ratio of effort in road races usually produces the best results, but you can only accomplish it if you continually apply pressure. Think of it as if you need to step slowly down on the accelerator to maintain an even speed. Marathons are different. You will usually slow down because of the depletion of glycogen stores.

Running the Race

The pace you fall into should match your physical preparation. You can be running a bit faster than your assessments, but if the pace is way over your head, be wary. On the other hand, don't be content to secure a comfortable place in the pack. Racing is the time for bravery. It's OK to let someone pull you along, but don't run haphazardly. At the beginning, stay well contained. Knowing the other runners doesn't help much. You'll end up with the right partner anyway. The best advice is to keep to your own plan but respond spontaneously. Trust your instincts. Feel when it is best to hang off the pace, when to move forward.

Early on, run steady and conserve energy. Knowing the place of transition from the start to the body of the race is a knowledge acquired only through racing experience. Let time pass. Be alert but go somewhat blank. Cerutty recommends a gaze set inches in front, slanted downward. Anything can happen. You may be running well and fall over. This happened to Ron Clarke once when he was running against John Landy. "Gentleman" John stopped and turned to inquire about Clarke's condition before continuing on, but this kind of spontaneous sportsmanship is rare in top-class competition.

You should run the body of the race in fresh or good swing. In this book you have been introduced to many new ways of running, and I hope you have tried them in your daily practices. The heat of competition can be the best place to practice. Try a shoulder breath, canter, conjure up a visualization. Imagining being pulled by a rope or carried by a large hand may provide just the right frame of mind. When becoming fatigued, exhale in a relaxed, prolonged breath.

As the race progresses, your place in the drama will unfold. You will begin feeling the discomfort of the pace. At some climactic moment all your concentration will be necessary to bring out your whole potential. Frank Shorter explains the courage of this moment: "You decide whether to go or not, afterwards, there is intensity but no pain." Once the mind turns over the switch, the body will follow.

The Finish

The basic rule for the last stage of a race is to have some idea about where you will begin your sprint. This is true for track as well as road races. Be decisive. A golden rule of racing is when you go . . . *go*. Don't play around. The jump may get you the decision even if you falter after passing. In a close race use the surge technique. The sprint form will help in a race of any distance. Once you are finished, keep walking. Use the candle breath to regain normal breathing. At times you will need to bend over to regain your breath. *Under no circumstances let anyone give you oxygen.* It could suffocate you. Put on your sweats. If you have time, lie down and go through the autogenic recovery routine. After long races, because of the prolonged silence there will be much bantering. Let yourself indulge but keep moving if you can. An excellent idea is to do a few shake-ups or to shuffle.

After the Race

Get a shower and satisfy your thirst. Even if you have drunk frequently during the race, you probably didn't satisfy all your body's needs. Electrolyte solutions are excellent. The stress is over, so whatever the outcome, let go and enjoy yourself. Good coaches know when to make themselves invisible. When things go badly a runner needs the coach's support, but he doesn't hang around to secure his own dose of the limelight. Better to walk off like the Lone Ranger into the sunset.

The day after the race is an excellent time for the runner to go for a long slow run. You may be a bit sore, but your ligaments and joints will be rested from the prerace rest. Review your training diary. Plan carefully for the future. A few quality races are better than a lot of mediocre ones. Roger Bannister ran the first four-minute mile at the end of a winter's training. Hungarian Sandor Iharos broke the 10,000-meter record after six months of training.

Don't race more than three times a month, except during a peaking cycle that may occur at the end of the year. Then every few days is all right, because afterward there will be a prolonged rest or light training. Remember, the sequence that ends in peak functioning brings happy, successful racing.

Glossary

absolute samadhi—meditation in which the state of no time, no space, and no causation is realized.

acceleration—run in which tempo is gradually increased.

accessory breathing—restricted breathing in which lungs do not fill to capacity because of tension.

acetyl-coA molecules—molecules that produce citrates or ketones from pyruvates.

acupuncture—massage technique which puts pressure on body's meridian points.

acupuncture needles—small needles used to puncture the body to activate body's meridian points.

advanced runner—person able to run a mile in 5½ to 7 minutes.

aerobic interval—distance at which heartbeat gets into the midpoint of the exercise heart range. This develops the runner's maximum oxygen consumption uptake.

aerobic metabolism—signifies the presence of ample oxygen at the cellular level.

aerobics—popular program, conceived by Dr. Kenneth Cooper, that measures maximum oxygen uptake.

aikido—Japanese art of self-defense that places emphasis on energy flow.

alpha block—a stimulant that breaks a meditator's production of alpha brain waves.

alpha brain wave pattern—brain wave pattern of 8–12 cycles per second that has a person vacillating between sleeping and total consciousness.

alveoli—the sites of oxygen-carbon dioxide exchange within the lungs.

amble—second phase of Cerutty's naturalistic running technique.

anaerobic intervals—gets the heartbeat near and/or over the high point of the exercise heart range, and breathing becomes predominantly anaerobic.

anaerobic metabolism—signifies that insufficient oxygen is available at the cellular level.

appliances—plastic or leather supports inside running shoes that realign the body.

autogenic recovery process—using autogenic training procedures to recover after a running workout.

autonomic nervous system—the sympathetic and parasympathetic divisions of the nervous system that control the functions of the heart, lungs, intestines, glands, and other internal organs and of the smooth muscles, blood vessels, and lymph vessels.

autonomic process—change that occurs automatically without our having to think about it.

bamboo stick—what Zen master hits meditator with to stimulate him when he dozes during meditation.

beginner—one who runs the mile in 10 to 15 minutes.

beta cycle—most active beta brain wave pattern (13–30 cycles per second), which is most suitable for analytical work.

bioentrainment—when two runners "flow" with each other.

biofeedback—name of method that uses a machine to give signals which tell meditator when he has brain wave patterns under voluntary control.

blowing out candle—breathing technique to achieve respiratory recovery.

body image meditation—guided fantasy that develops awareness of physical identity.

breathing coordination—name of respiratory method developed by Carl Stough.

breathing cycle—entire sequence of exhalation and inhalation.

calisthenics—light gymnastics exercises derived from German military tradition.

calling the distance—technique to achieve fartlek training.

canter—asymmetrical gait in Cerutty's naturalistic running.

carbon dioxide tension—excess build-up of carbon dioxide in the bloodstream due to acceleration of ATP's.

cardiac threshold—heartbeat at which an individual's exercise is providing the training effect. Beginning of exercise heart change.

ch'an—Chinese word for "meditation."

chant—word or phrase, repeated verbally or silently, that promotes an altered state of consciousness.

chiropractic—healing by manipulation of spine.

classical interval school—specific number of intervals, each at a predetermined specific time and distance, and each with a specific recovery period between end of interval and beginning of another.

competitive rank—runner able to run faster than a 4:40 mile or equivalent.

conditioning—occurs through gradual adaptation to stress.

creatine phosphate—a small reserve of quick energy stored in the muscles.

crystalline moments—situations in which activities deliver peak experiences.

delta—deep sleep or dreaming state.

detached awareness—consciousness sought in Zen meditation.

diastolic pressure—the pressure during relaxation of heart.

EKG test—a readout diagnosis of heart rhythm.

electroencephalogram (EEG)—graph that measures brain-wave patterns.

electrolytes—ions such as sodium, potassium, calcium, and magnesium lost through sweating.

electron transfer system—a chain of molecules that are oxidized during aerobic metabolism.

energy body—name given to field of energy or self directly outside the physical person.

energy transfer—giving of personal power to another.

epinephrine—secreted from sympathetic nervous system; many consider it the cause of runner's high.

Esalen Institute—grandfather institution that led to the human potentials movement.

Esalen Sports Center—special section of Esalen Institute devoted to mind-body approach to running. Mike Spino is director.

exceptional rank—person able to run the mile between 4:40 and 5:30.

exercise heart range—graph of specific beats of heart per minute which serves as an indicator of the optimum level of stress you need to subject your body to in order to cause a positive physical adaptation.

excitatory transmitter—chemical transmission of thoughts that are immediately conscious.

fartlek—Swedish term for "speed play," i.e., alternating slower and faster running.

Finnish breathing system—practice of synchronizing breath and steps.

fitness index—Dr. George Sheehan's recommendation as way to check daily state of health.

fresh swing tempo—swing gait between 15 and 50 percent effort.

full lung aeration—Cerutty's term for getting full use of lung capacity.

gait—how you run.

gallop—asymmetrical final and fastest gait of naturalistic Cerutty running.

glucose—one of simple sugars into which carbohydrates must be broken down before absorption into bloodstream can occur.

glycogen—chief storage carbohydrate burned up while running.

glycolysis—the mainstay of anaerobic metabolism; produces two ATP molecules.

good speed—variation in gait for acceleration or recovery.

good swing tempo—swing gait between 50 and 80 percent effort.

guided fantasy—story line that has universal application, told to people in meditation.

hemoglobin—iron-rich substance in red blood cells that transports oxygen and carbon dioxide.

hypothalamus—possible control mechanism for fight-or-flight mechanism.

inhibitory transmitter—chemical impulse from brain that does not become conscious.

intermediate rank—person who can run a mile in seven to ten minutes.

intervals—planned runs with specific rest periods.

junction point—spot at which runner changes from one gait and tempo to another.

kensho—word for "enlightenment."

ketosis—scientists' term for the "wall" in a marathon.

Krebs cycle—name of the process combining oxygen with citrates of acetyl-coA molecules that produces 38 molecules of ATP.

lactate—waste material that is end product of anaerobic metabolism.

lactovegetarian—vegetarian diet which includes fish and poultry but not red meat.

left side of brain—where rational, logical thought process occurs.

levitate—to rise in air and float in defiance of gravity.

LFD—long fast distance running.

long continuous distance—running long distances at steady pace.

long-distance running—racing distances from 3 to 10 miles.

lung-gom runners—legendary ultralong-distance runners of Tibet.

mantra—usually Sanskrit word repeated verbally or nonverbally that slows down flow of thoughts.

maximum breathing capacity—greatest number of liters of air that can be processed each minute.

maximum heart range—85 to 100 percent of possible heartbeats per minute.

maximum oxygen uptake—the amount of air consumed while doing maximum work.

mental practice—training of the mind to aid in physical activity.

metabolic ratio—proportion of aerobic to anaerobic metabolism.

metabolism—the chemical and physical process continually going on in living organisms and cells, comprising those by which assimilated foods are built into protoplasm and those by which protoplasm is used and broken down into simpler substances or waste matter, with the release of energy for all vital processes.

middle distance—races for 0.5 to 3 miles.

mitochondria—powerhouse of the cell where Krebs cycle and electron transfer system take place.

moving visualizations—having pictures in the mind while running.

myoglobin—iron-rich protein permanently fixed in the cell.

naturalistic running—Cerutty's technique in which you learn to run like an animal.

neurons—nerve cells in brain that are constantly processing information.

osteopathy—medical system in which doctor specializes in manipulation that realigns bone and muscle.

oxygen consumption—amount of oxygen that is utilized by metabolism of the cells.

oxygen transport system—cardiovascular system of heart, veins, arteries, capillaries, and blood plasma that gets oxygen from lungs to muscles.

pain one—minor pain.

pain two—severe pain.

peak experience—situation in which you discover your fullest self.

percentage of maximum oxygen consumption—most accurate measurement of fitness while running middle to ultralong distances.

perspiration—the most efficient heat reduction mechanism.

pH balance—measurement of alkaline versus acid level in the blood.

podiatrists—foot doctors who have become specialists in treating running injuries.

Portsea—location of Cerutty's training camp in Australia.

positive mental attitude—meditator's passive stance.

power run—resistance exercise done on flat surface.

primary tank—name given diaphragm area during breathing.

progressive relaxation—technique of tightening and loosening muscles to promote relaxation, developed by Edmund Jacobsen.

psychic dependency—relying on another person or belief system to maintain personality and equilibrium.

psychic self-regulation—Soviet-founded combination of mental practices to improve physical performance through mental training.

psychic survival—living without spiritual death.

psychosomatic pain—physical pain that has an emotional base.

pyruvates—molecules of citrates or ketones besides the two ATPs that are produced in glycolysis.

rank—designates time in the mile run.

recovery period—the time in which the heart returns to a lower rate.

recreational runner—person who runs a mile in more than 4:40.

relaxation—key to success in any activity.

repetition interval—specific run which gets heart to maximum exertion level and depths of anaerobic metabolism.

resistance training—training by use of an uphill grade.

resting pulse—number of beats per minute of heart at rest. Normally 10 to 15 beats either side of 72.

right side of brain—where intuitive, instinctive thoughts occur.

ritual—preparation for a sacred rite.

Royal Canadian Air Force exercises—system that combines calisthenic-type exercises and cardiorespiratory workouts.

runner's high—general name given to bliss state achieved through running.

runner's irony—an attitude that forms when a runner is no longer a beginner.

running—another name could be "moving meditation."

samadhi—ultimate consciousness of pure bliss.

Sanskrit—language of India, now reserved for sacred matters.

satori—state of spiritual enlightenment in Zen.

second wind—revitalization of energy during a run.

secondary tank—term given chest area in respiration.

sesshin—Zen practice of long duration that combines various forms of meditation.

set—a number of intervals grouped together in order to accomplish a specific physiological purpose.

shag interval—interval run before full recovery.

shoulder breathing—relaxation breathing technique that uses lift of shoulder to fully fill lungs.

shuffle—slowest gait; below 15 percent effort.

skip and shake-up—running warm-up technique.

soft eyes—technique for keeping mental pictures in head while moving about.

sprint—85 to 100 percent effort.

sprint form process—technique of learning proper sprinting form.

stretch-up—reaching overhead to begin naturalistic running.

stroke volume—amount of blood pumped from the heart with each beat.

structural integration—Ida Rolf's name for deep tissue massage.

systolic pressure—peak pressure within blood vessels when the heart is contracting.

tempo—how fast you run.

theta—sleep.

tidal breathing—breathing technique using inhaled air for forward propulsion.

tiger balm—a Chinese liniment.

time assessment—practice race to accomplish specific physiological task.

training sequence—a series of workouts with a specific goal.

trophotropic response—a protective mechanism in hypothalamus that promotes restorative process (relates to physiologic changes measured in meditation).

ultralong distances—runs of over 10 miles.

unstressing—in meditation, indicates the release of stress on the level of nerve and muscle.

visualization—creating a preplanned image in the mind while running.

vital capacities—reasearch measurements that determine fitness.

workshop—gathering of people to learn about method, philosophy, technique, and so on, over a defined period of time.

zazen—name given to meditation session in Zen.

Zen koan—Zen puzzle.

Zen meditation—Japanese form of meditation; key to utilizing the mind during running.

Index

Acceleration, 121

Acetyl-CoA, 98–99

Actionade, 110

Adenosine triphosphate (ATP), 95–97, 98, 99, 101, 103, 104, 105, 106, 108, 109, 111, 113

Aerobic capacity, 99

Aerobic intervals, 139

Aerobic vs. anaerobic metabolism, 97

Aerobics (Cooper), 105

Aikido, 42

Alpha brain waves, 16, 20

Amble, naturalistic, 131

Anaerobic vs. aerobic metabolism, 97

Anaerobic intervals, 139

Anderson, Arne, 5

Anderson, Aobert, 70

ATP. *See* Adenosine triphosphate

Bannister, Roger, 3, 7, 12, 125, 195

Benson, Herbert, 16

Billinger, Bill, 138

Blowing out the candle technique, 64

Body image meditation, 50–51

Bodymind (Dychtwald), 70

Boredom, 36–41

Breathing
 basics of, 60–61
 exercises, 61, 62–69
 techniques, 8
 and walking, 63–64
 in Zen meditation, 29–30

Burleson, Dyrol, 123

"Burning" energy, 109

Canter, naturalistic, 134–36

Carbohydrates, 95, 108, 111

Carbon dioxide, 101

Carbon dioxide tension, 101

Carbon monoxide, 107

Cerutty, Percy, 7, 10, 12, 28, 61, 62, 123, 125, 129, 131, 132, 135, 148, 156, 183, 189, 193, 194

Cicero, 36
Clarke, Ron, 194
Cooling down, 109–10
Cooper, Kenneth, 102, 105
Corbitt, Ted, 181
Costill, David, 106, 190
CP. *See* Creatine phosphate
Cramps, 110
Creatine phosphate (CP), 96, 104

Dawes, Ron, 13
Dehydration, 109
Deines, Bob, 187
Diet for runners, 183–84, 190–191
Doherty, J. Kenneth, 3
Dychtwald, Kenneth, 70

Elliott, Herb, 7–9, 10, 12, 27, 28, 40, 131, 156, 183
Emmerton, Bill, 10, 116
Energy production in the cell, 95–96
    oxygen and, 95–101, 103, 105, 106–07
Environments for running, 182
ERG, 110, 183
Esalen Sports Center, 2, 187
Evans, Lee, 126, 190

Fartlek training, 4, 10, 143–44
    visualization in, 58
    workouts, 161
Flight response, 17
Frederick, E. C., 105
Fresh swing, 118
Fresh swing tempo, 6

Gait, *See also specific gaits,* 115
Gallop, naturalistic, 136–37
Garrison, Jim, 6
Gatorade, 110, 183
Getting Straight, 26
Glucose, 96

Glycogen, 104, 108
Glycolysis, 96, 97, 98, 104, 111
Golden Mile, The (Elliott), 40
Good speed, 120
Good swing, 119–20
Good swing tempo, 6
Gould, Elliott, 26
Guided fantasies, 45–50

Haegg, Gunder, 5
Hall Circuit, 9
Harbig, Rudolf, 4
Hard speed, 6
Hard swing tempo, 6
Health and running, 185–86
Heart, 101–03
Heart rate, 102
Hemery, David, 174
Hemoglobin, 100, 103, 107
Henderson, Joe, 185
Holmer, Gosta, 4
Human Movement Potential (Swigart), 58
Huxley, Aldous, 30
Hypothalamus, 17

Igloi, Mihaly, 5–7, 12, 123, 138, 148
Iharos, Sandor, 5, 195
International Meditation Society, 15
Interval training, 5–7, 10, 107, 115, 138–39
    aerobic, 139
    anaerobic, 139
    repetition, 140
    shag, 139
    sprinting, 141–42
    value of, 140–41
    visualization in, 58
    workouts, 158–59, 168–69

Jipcho, Ben, 190
Jogging, 174

Jones, John Paul, 4
Junction point, 121

Keats, John, 32
Ketosis, 108
Kidd, Bruce, 131
Krebs cycle, 98–99, 112
Kuts, Vladimir, 193

Lactic acid, 104
Landy, John, 7, 194
Larrieu, Francie, 146
LCD. *See* Long continuous distance running
Leonard, George, 43, 187
Lewis, A. J., 44
Lombardi, Vince, 6
Long continuous distance running (LCD), 115, 137. *See also* Marathon
workouts, 157–58, 162–63
LCD training, 106–07
Lung-gom, 10–11, 34, 58
Lydiard, Arthur, 9–10, 69, 137, 148, 190

Marathon, 165, 169–77
training for, 9–10
Maximum oxygen capacity, 106
Meditation, 11
body image, 51–55
running and, 10–11, 15–41
transcendental, 15, 19
Zen, 19–24
Meditation in Action (Chogyam Trungpa), 20
Metabolism
aerobic, 98–100
anaerobic, 97–98
Middle-distance running, 165–168
Miling, 165
Miller, Martin, 187
Mitochondria, 112
MOC. *See* Maximum oxygen capacity

Morehouse, Laurence, 114, 184
Murphy, Michael, 32, 56, 181, 187
Murphy's law, 149
Myoglobin, 100, 107, 112

Norepinephrine, 18
Nurmi, Paavo, 4

Oxygen, 98–100, 103, 106
consumption of, 20, 106
energy production and, 98–101

Pain, Zen meditation and, 30–36
Perspiration, 109
Physiology. *See also specific organs*
of relaxation, 17–18
running and, 93–113
training and, 110–13
Pirsig, Robert, 24
Plateaus, 187–88
Power run, 129–30
Protein, 95
PSR Foundation, 44
Psychology, 13–24
Pyruvic acid, 98

Racing, 188–95
Relaxation, 17–18
visualization and, 42–43
Relaxation Response, The (Benson), 16
Repetition intervals, 140
Resistance running, 142–43
Resistance training, 115
workouts, 159–60
Rockne, Knute, 9
Roszavolgy, Istvan, 5
Runner's high, 13, 26
"Runners' punch," 110
Runners World (magazine), 185

Running. *See also* Sprinting; Shuffle
 boredom in, 36–38
 breathing techniques in, 8, 29–30, 60–61
 diet for, 183–85
 environments, 182
 equipment, 181–82
 meditation and, 11, 15–41
 mental aspects of, 1–11, 18–19, 93–94
 naturalistic, 130–31
 pain and, 30–34
 physiology of, 93–113
 psychology of, 13–24
 smoking and, 107
 training program for, 5–10, 114–80
 visualization in, 34–59
 weather and, 182–83
Running with Cerutty, 129
Running Home (Spiro), 56
Running partners, 187
Running sesshin, 55–58

Samadhi, 22, 30
Satori, 30
Second wind, 93, 104
Sekida, Katsuki, 23
Shag, 169
Shag intervals, 139
Sheehan, George, 185
Shorter, Frank, 194
Shoulder breathing, 67–69
Shuffle, 10, 116–18
Silent Pulse, The (Leonard), 187
Skip shake-up, 121–23
Smoking, 107
Snell, Peter, 9, 125, 190
So You Want to be a Sprinter, (Winters), 178
"Soft eyes" technique, 56
Speed play. *See* Fartlek training
Speed workouts, 160–61

Sprinting, *See also* Running. 5, 126–29, 174–78
Standing visualization, 42–43
Stationary breath holding, 64
Stones, Dwight, 146
Stough, Carl, 63
Stretching, 69–71
 exercises, 71–92
Stretch-up, naturalistic, 131
Supine breathing, 63
Surge, 123–25

Tabori, Laszio, 5
Tidal breathing, 64–67
TM. *See* Transcendental meditation
Total Fitness (Morehouse), 114
Training, 3–12, 114–42
 Fartlek, 4, 10, 161–62
 interval, 4–9, 10, 115, 138–142
 long continuous distance, 107, 115, 137–39, 157–158, 162–63
 marathon, 165, 169–76
 middle-distance, 165–68
 physiology and, 110–13
 resistance, 115, 159–60
 shuffle, 10, 116–18
 six-week program, 145–80
Transcendental meditation (TM), 15–16, 19–20. *See also* Zen meditation
Trot, naturalistic, 132–34
Trungpa, Chogyam, 20
Tucker, Ben, 126

Visualization, 34–41
 exercises, 42
 relaxation by, 40–41
 standing, 42–43
Vitamins, 184–85

"Wall," 93–94, 107–09
Wayne, Ron, 171

Weather and running, 182–83
Weight lifting, 186
Winters, Bud, 126, 178

Yeats, W. B., 27
Yoga meditations, vs. Zen meditations, 20–21
Yogi, Maharishi Mahesh, 15

Zatopek, Emil, 64, 131
Zazen. *See* Zen meditation
Zen and the Art of Motorcycle Maintenance (Pirsig), 24

Zen meditation, 19–24. *See also* Transcendental meditation
breathing and, 29–30
pain and, 30–34
running and, 25–41
yoga vs., 21
Zen Training, Methods and Philosophy, 23
Zen walk, 56–57

ABOUT THE AUTHORS

MIKE SPINO is director of the well-known Esalen Sports Center in Big Sur, California. With Michael Murphy, co-founder of the Esalen Institute (and its president for twelve years), Spino has put together a unique four-day session for runners at the plush Princess Tower Hotel in the Bahamas—a program which stresses the unity of mind, emotion, body and spirit in athletic activity. Spino has trained with some of the foremost track coaches of the last fifty years and has adapted their methods in his own workshops. Spino is the author of *Beyond Jogging* and *Running Home: The Body/Mind Family Fitness.*

A graduate of the University of California at Berkeley, JEFFREY EARL WARREN has written newspaper columns, television commercials and comedy shows, and magazine articles. He has taught creative writing and is presently working on a novel.

BE A WINNER
IN THE RACE FOR
FITNESS

These physical fitness titles give every member of the family the guidance they need for getting in shape and keeping fit. Choose the program most suited to you whether it be yoga, jogging, or an exercise routine. You'll feel better for it.

☐	12261	**DR. SHEEHAN ON RUNNING** George A. Sheehan	$2.25
☐	12382	**GETTING STRONG** Kathryn Lance	$2.50
☐	12289	**RUNNING FOR HEALTH AND BEAUTY** Kathryn Lance	$2.25
☐	11166	**JAZZERCISE** Missett & Meilach	$1.95
☐	13061	**LILIAS, YOGA AND YOU** Lilias Folan	$2.25
☐	12546	**NICOLE RONSARD'S NO-EXCUSE** **EXERCISE GUIDE** Nicole Ronsard	$1.95
☐	12540	**AEROBICS** Kenneth H. Cooper	$2.25
☐	12468	**AEROBICS FOR WOMEN** Cooper & Cooper	$2.25
☐	11902	**THE AEROBICS WAY** Kenneth H. Cooper	$2.50
☐	12360	**THE NEW AEROBICS** Kenneth H. Cooper	$2.25
☐	12322	**CELLULITE** Nicole Ronsard	$1.95
☐	11282	**THE ALEXANDER TECHNIQUE** Sara Barker	$1.95
☐	11246	**INTRODUCTION TO YOGA** Richard Hittleman	$1.95
☐	11976	**YOGA 28 DAY EXERCISE PLAN** Richard Hittleman	$2.25

Buy them at your local bookstore or use this handy coupon for ordering:

Bantam Book Catalog

Here's your up-to-the-minute listing of over 1,400 titles by your favorite authors.

This illustrated, large format catalog gives a description of each title. For your convenience, it is divided into categories in fiction and non-fiction—gothics, science fiction, westerns, mysteries, cookbooks, mysticism and occult, biographies, history, family living, health, psychology, art.

So don't delay—take advantage of this special opportunity to increase your reading pleasure.

Just send us your name and address and 50¢ (to help defray postage and handling costs).